OXFORD MEDICAL PUBLICATIONS

Constipation in Childhood

CONSTIPATION IN CHILDHOOD

GRAHAM CLAYDEN

Reader in Paediatrics,
United Medical and Dental School
of Guy's and St Thomas' Hospitals

and

ULFUR AGNARSSON

Honorary Lecturer, King's College Hospital, and
Research Fellow, Hospital for Sick Children
Great Ormond Street and Queen Elizabeth Hospital

OXFORD   NEW YORK   TOKYO
OXFORD UNIVERSITY PRESS
1991

Oxford University Press, Walton Street, Oxford OX2 6DP

Oxford New York Toronto
Delhi Bombay Calcutta Madras Karachi
Petaling Jaya Singapore Hong Kong Tokyo
Nairobi Dar es Salaam Cape Town
Melbourne Auckland

and associated companies in
Berlin Ibadan

Oxford is a trade mark of Oxford University Press

Published in the United States
by Oxford University Press, New York

© Graham Clayden and Ulfur Agnarsson, 1991

British Library Cataloguing-in-Publication Data
Clayden, Graham
Constipation in childhood.
1. Children. Constipation
I. Title II. Agnarsson, Ulfur
618.923428
ISBN 0–19–262044–4
ISBN 0–19–262027–4 (pbk)

Library of Congress Cataloging in Publication Data
Clayden, Graham.
Constipation in childhood / Graham Clayden, Ulfur Agnarsson.
Includes bibliographical references.
Includes index.
1. Constipation in children. I. Agnarsson, Ulfur. II. Title.
[DNLM: 1. Constipation—in infancy & childhood. WI 409 C622c]
RJ456.C76C58 1991   618.92' 3428—dc20   90-7918
ISBN 0–19–262044–4
ISBN 0–19–262027–4 (pbk)

Phototypeset by Dobbie Typesetting Service, Tavistock, Devon

Printed in Great Britain by
Bookcraft (Bath) Ltd
Midsomer Norton, Avon

Preface

Constipation in childhood poses a number of difficult questions. Which child will need further investigation? Is this a simple management problem where advice on increasing fluid intake and dietary fibre will suffice? What is the pathophysiology of the megarectum? Why are the child and family behaving in this way? How effective and safe are laxatives in childhood? What are the indications for surgical treatment?

This book goes some way to answering these and other questions. It should arm the doctor managing or co-ordinating the treatment with background knowledge, thus helping the professionals to form a concept of the particular weave of factors involved in the evolution and persistence of the individual child's problem. This concept assists communication with the child and family, and between professionals. So often treatment regimes are started without this initial analysis and the direction is wrong from the outset. It is as damaging for a child with constipation provoked by severe anal pain to be given suppositories as it is for a child with a structural abnormality to be persuaded by a professional that they can open their bowels when they cannot, however much they try.

The use of laxatives is another area where there is confusion. The commonly used laxatives are reviewed and the indications listed. Management algorithms are given and the decision points discussed in the text.

This book should help the paediatrician in the important role of communicator and co-ordinator. It should help the surgeon and psychiatrist or psychologist to understand each others' roles. It should help the family doctor who must decide which of the large number of infants with minor problems might go on to develop chronic constipation, and therefore, need to be referred before parental confidence is damaged.

London   G.C.
October, 1990   U.A.

Contents

1. Introduction

Although mild constipation is very common in childhood, when it is chronic or relapsing the child and the family face very distressing problems, which are sometimes underestimated by their professional helpers. This may lead to a denial of the importance of the symptoms and a delay in the planning of an effective strategy to help. A delay of this type may allow the development of vicious circles in the physiology of the anorectum as well as in the child's development and the family psychology. There has been considerable debate on the relative roles of the organic and psychogenic elements in the causes and persistence of bowel difficulty. Some of the confusion in the medical literature has arisen as a result of a failure to agree on a common set of definitions. Throughout this book the following definitions are used:

Constipation Difficulty or delay in the passage of stools (not a description of the hardness of the stool, although this is often but not always associated).

Soiling Involuntary passage of fluid or semi-solid stool into the clothing (usually as a result of overflow from a faecally loaded rectum).

Encopresis Passage of a normal stool into socially inappropriate places (including clothing).

CONSTIPATION IN HISTORY

The evolution of man as a social animal was made possible, in part, by the development of faecal continence. There was probably an enormous survival advantage in avoiding leaving a faecal trail when predators were about. Communal living was probably protected from outbreaks of infective diarrhoea when it was possible to separate defaecation and feeding spatially. The anatomical and physiological adaptations made to achieve this have taken their toll.

From the earliest recorded medical advice, great care was taken to ensure regularity of defaecation. The ancient Egyptians recommended weekly enemata to ensure complete evacuation of faecal residue (Herodotus, Book II, 77). Soranus recommended routine rectal examinations in the new-born to break down any residual anorectal membrane and allow the free passage of faeces.[1]

Nearly all treatises on medicine had several remedies to aid evacuation of the faeces using a variety of medications, many of which are active according to modern analysis. It has always been assumed that the retention of faeces leads to some deleterious effect by releasing harmful substances into the body. This is very eloquently described by Harris (translated by John Martyn in 1742) in his *A treatise of the acute diseases of infants*.[2]

'But that the purging, tho' it is not reckoned among the Arcana of Physick, and owes hardly anything to the wonders of Chymistry, is indeed the Principle of all helps, which is the fruitful invention of curious men ever discovered, I am persuaded to believe chiefly for this reason, that hardly anyone has a firm State of Health, or can keep himself in good order, unless his body be moderately open every day by natural purging; which natural purging is almost as necessary to sustain life, and preserve the Health of the Body, as our own daily Meat and Drink is to the nourishment of it. Nor does the Method of Living more require, that the better and more juice part of the food should be transmitted through the lacteal veins, to afford due Nourishment to the Body, than the thicker and worse part of it, which being too long retained sends up noxious, and in a manner venomous steams, should be expelled from the body through the common sink, either by Nature or Art. And, indeed, purging has justly acquired such Honour to itself, that common custom has dignified that operation alone with the Name of Physick.'

We hope to convey some of Walter Harris's enthusiasm for the subject in this book, even if we fail to match John Martyn's literary flair, and help the reader to understand the relevant parts of Nature and to acquire some of the attributes of the Art.

The control of faecal continence and the social pressures to conform appear to run together. This was suggested by the work on the North American Indian tribes by Whiting and Child.[3] They describe the association of vigorous faecal continence training in early childhood with savage behaviour in the adults, and vice versa.

Fredick Ruysch of Amsterdam seems to have been the first to describe very serious constipation when he described the finding of a grossly dilated colon in a five-year old girl who had died; 'Enormis intestinis coli dilatatis'. Harald Hirschsprung[4] described two fatal cases of megacolon in 1887, but it was 1949[5] before the aganglionic, narrow distal segment of the bowel was shown to be the cause of this, the most serious form of obstructive constipation, although Karl Tittel[6] had suggested this as early as 1901. When this clinical entity was accepted as a cause of severe constipation, all other cases were considered to be psychogenic and a plethora of papers strengthened this view. In the early 1960s support was gathering for a fairer recognition of both physical and psychological causes for constipation and soiling. Unfortunately, the pendulum swung too far and medical authorities became partisan in their support for either a physical or psychological cause.

Gradually it has become accepted that constipation and overflow faecal soiling are the result of a pathological system which involves both physical and psychological factors. Bowel problems, especially those associated with the shame and rejection of faecal incontinence, inevitably lead to stresses in the individual and the family, whatever the original physical cause. Similarly, stress and emotional disturbance have an effect on the function of the bowels as most people can recall from their own experience before tests or examinations.

Historically, the gradual change in perception of the clinical entity of constipation and overflow has mirrored the broader acceptance of the link between the physical and the psychological at all ages in medicine and the need for a multidisciplinary effort to help.

References

1. Soranus (1965). *Gynaecology*, Bk. 2, ch. 13, p. 83–4, (trans. O. Temkin). Johns Hopkins Press, Baltimore.
2. Harris W. (1742). *A treatise of the acute diseases of infants*. Royal College of Physicians, London.
3. Whiting, J. W. and Child, I. L. (1953). *Child training and personality*. Yale University Press, New Haven.
4. Hirschsprung, H. (1887). Constipation in the newborn due to dilatation and hypertrophy of the colon. *Jahrb. Kinderheilk.* 27, 1–7. [In German.]
5. Bodian, M., Stephens, F. D., and Ward, B. C. H. (1949). Hirschsprung's disease and idiopathic megacolon. *Lancet* i, 6–11.
6. Tittel, K. (1901). Uber eine angeboerene Missbildung des Dietdarmes. *Wiener Klin. Woch.* 39, 903–7.

DESIGN OF THIS BOOK

This book is designed to supply the reader with sufficient background basic science about the often neglected area of the anorectum, in order to understand the rationale behind the management strategies of the more common clinical problems.

Following the section on the anatomy and embryology of the gut, there is a review of the physiology of faecal continence and defaecation. This leads on to chapters on the presentation of these problems at different ages, the special problems of children with other disabilities, and then the management schemes. Details of treatments and medications are followed by descriptions and evaluations of different investigative procedures and surgical treatments. The role of psychological treatments of different types is reviewed in outline. The concluding section of the book is a specimen explanatory booklet designed for the average, bright 10-year old, which readers can adapt to their own use.

2. Scientific background

ANATOMY

The anal canal measures 2.5–4.0 cm in length (Fig. 1).[1] It is the area between the anal verge and the junction of the stratified cuboidal and columnar epithelium (dentate line).[2] It is lined by squamous epithelium in the lower anal canal but changes to stratified cuboidal and, finally, columnar epithelium higher up. High in the anal canal the mucosa is thrown into four to six major folds with fewer, minor folds between.

The smooth muscle of the internal anal sphincter is continuous with, and is formed by, the inner circular muscle of the rectum. It becomes more prominent low in the anal canal. It is approximately 3 cm long and 5 mm thick.[3] It is made up of two distinct parts which function together as one unit. They are separated by muscle fibres of the puboanalis muscle and the anterior sacrococcygeal ligament, which together insert into the dermis of the anal skin just below the mucocutaneous junction. Both sympathetic and parasympathetic nerves innervate the internal sphincter. The parasympathetic nerves originate in the sacral plexus and they reduce the sphincter tone, while the sympathetic nerves form the thoracolumbar plexus increase anal tone.[4]

The external anal sphincter is a striated muscle and consists of a deep and a superficial part. It surrounds the anal orifice. It is innervated by rami of the pudendal and perineal nerves, which originate from sacral roots 2–4.[5] The sphincter is also supplied by local intramural purinergic nerves, which are neither sympathetic nor parasympathetic, and these nerves mediate the relaxation response during rectal distension.[4]

The pelvic floor muscles consist of the levator ani muscle group one part of which, the puborectal muscle, forms a sling around the anorectal junction. This creates an angle between the anus and the rectum, the anorectal angle, which is

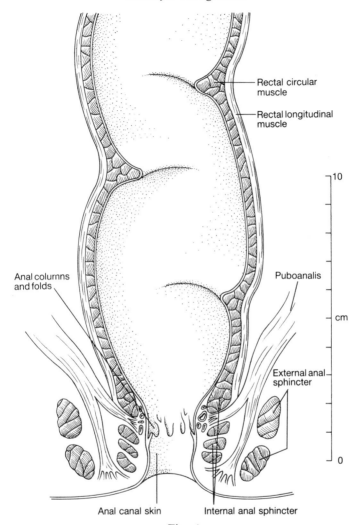

Rectal circular muscle

Rectal longitudinal muscle

10

Anal columns and folds

Puboanalis

cm

External anal sphincter

0

Anal canal skin

Internal anal sphincter

Fig. 1

80–90 degrees at rest and during defaecation is more obtuse, at 100–105 degrees.[6] Above the levator ani the highest part of the anal canal joins the rectum. The dissected rectum measures 12.5 cm in the adult. When empty its walls collapse and so it remains until just before defaecation, when it fills. It is an extremely distensible organ.

PHYSIOLOGY OF ANAL CONTINENCE

Knowledge of the physiology of continence is an important foundation for a full understanding of the disturbances leading to constipation and soiling in children.

Continence is achieved by the adaptive compliance of the colon with the retentive mechanism of the anorectum. Normally, the distal rectum is empty and collapsed.[7] The simple anatomical impedance to the descending faecal mass occurs because the distal end of the gastrointestinal tract is not a straight tube. The angulations in the aptly named sigmoid colon and the spiral folds (valves of Houston) impede the caudal faecal movement. Another important kink which assists continence is the 80° angle between the axis of the rectum and the axis of the anal canal.[8] This helpful kink is maintained by the puboanal sling, a part of the puborectalis muscle in association with the external anal sphincter.[9,10] Apart from merely causing a circuitous route for the stool, these angulations help in maintaining continence during sudden rises in intra-abdominal pressure such as sneezing, laughing, and postural change. This extraluminal, intra-abdominal pressure collapses the lumen in a 'flap valve'[11] and a 'flutter valve'[8] manner. The flattening of the angulations produces the 'flap valve' and the flattening of the normally collapsed, slit-like anorectum produces the 'flutter valve'. Intraluminal pressure will open the flutter valve in the same way as air blown through a length of soft latex-rubber tubing. The longitudinal mucosal folds in the anus also contribute to continence of semi-solid or fluid faeces by the way they fold together, even when the internal sphincter partially relaxes.

The anal sphincters play an important role in maintaining continence and both the voluntary external sphincter and the involuntary internal sphincter have a resting tone. This is an unusual quality for a striated muscle that, fortunately, also persists during sleep. However, the external sphincter does fatigue when maximally contracted, after about 50 seconds in adults[12] and about 30 seconds in children. This is important to remember when considering whether constipation due to deliberate withholding of faeces is possible in every child or just those with a physical predisposition.

The internal sphincter has a rhythmical fluctuation in anal tone, normally around 30–40 mmHg. This is sufficient to protect against soiling unless the muscle is inhibited via the myenteric plexus and the recto-anal reflex, when the rectum is distended or contracting.

The sensory innervation from the lower end of the bowel is very important in maintaining continence. The rectum has only skein-like stretch receptors which have an increasing sensitivity the more distal they are sited. The anal canal is richly endowed with sensory receptors for most modalities of sensation.[13] These receptors, together with the configuration of the anal mucosal folds, allow us to distinguish between flatus, fluid, and faeces, before it is too late.

Continence in children develops gradually when

(1) they recognize the sensation of rectal filling (via the stretch receptors);

(2) they realize that it is not socially accepted to defaecate immediately (following effective pot training);

(3) they impede the descent of the stool (by contracting the puboanal sling and external anal sphincter);

(4) they temporarily contain the stool in the upper rectum;

(5) they reinforce the contraction of these continence muscles each time the rectum contracts, sensation is produced, and the internal anal sphincter relaxes to allow the descent into the very sensitive upper anal canal.

Defaecation then occurs when the child has found a convenient refuge to relieve the increasing sense of urgency and rectal discomfort.

PHYSIOLOGY OF DEFAECATION

The defaecation sequence can be conveniently summarized as follows.

- filling of the rectum by colonic action;
- distension of the rectum and rectal contraction in response to this;
- sensation of the desire to defaecate, increasing in intensity as stool descends;
- descent of pelvic floor and relaxation of puboanalis, thus straightening the anorectum;
- inhibition of the internal sphincter and shortening of the anal canal;
- descent of the stool on to the sensory zone in the anal canal;
- increase in rectal pressure as external sphincter contracts initially;
- increase in sensation and intensity of rectal waves;
- urgent desire to defaecate and external sphincter fatigue;
- complete inhibition of the internal sphincter;
- glottic closure, Valsalva manoeuvre leading to increase in intra-abdominal pressure with the stool filling the anorectum;
- faecal expulsion, external sphincter contracts and internal sphincter exhibits closing activity as rectal distension ceases;
- a child experiences relief from the intensity of the urgent desire to defaecate;
- pleasure reinforced by parental acclaim.

Some further details of this process will help in understanding the pathophysiology of constipation.

Rectal filling

This depends on the motility in the colon, the role of which is to impede the flow of the faecal contents and to reabsorb water. If colonic activity is diminished it acts as a virtual drain-pipe leading to diarrhoea. Babies demonstrate the gastrocolic reflex very clearly even allowing a number of mothers to be quite successful initially in establishing a reliable system of catching the stool in a pot following a feed.

Reflex colonic filling of the rectum initiates a contraction of the rectal smooth muscles[14] and also promotes contractions in the right colon (rectocolic reflex).[15] Constipation of the non-megarectum type can be caused by hypermotility of the colon[16] illustrating the non-propulsive nature of most of the colonic waves.[17,18] Constipation of this type is more common in adults and in late-onset constipation in older children and adolescents.

The effects of emotion on colonic motility help to explain some of the physiological problems in encopresis. Hyper-motility is associated with anger, resentment, and hostility; hypomotility with depression; and some increase with cheerfulness.[19,20]

Rectal distension

As the rectum distends, the stretch receptors in its walls are activated, and as the stool descends even more receptors become involved and so sensation increases. There is an automatic reflex inhibition of the internal anal sphincter in response to rectal distension—the anorectal reflex.[14,21-24] This inhibition occurs in two phases. First, there is a sudden drop in pressure which inversely mirrors the rectal contraction. Secondly, there is a more sustained reduction in the squeeze pressure in the anal canal with increasing degree of rectal distension. When the initial inhibitory trough is matched in its degree of reduction in anal pressure by the sustained inhibition, the stool moves caudally, the sensation increases, and defaecation is obligatory. This inhibition is mediated by the myenteric nerves and so is absent in Hirschsprung's disease, leading to obstructive constipation. In children with massive megarectum, a very large volume of stool is required to produce complete and sustained internal sphincter inhibition, thus leading to the infrequent passage of massive stools with overflow faecal soiling seeping out following the initial inhibitory troughs. In these children the faecal mass may be so large that the rectum cannot propel the mass through the anus or the bony pelvis. It is possible to see complete inhibition (gaping) or temporary inhibitions (reflex anal dilatation) on anal inspection, depending on the degree of rectal faecal loading.

Rectal sensation

Rectal discomfort is probably the signal which both warns and motivates us to stop our current activity and search for a convenient place in which to defaecate in private. The sensation is mainly produced by the distending rectum activating the stretch receptors in its wall. Thus, the larger the rectum the more distension is required to produce the sensation of urgency or discomfort. In a child with a congenitally large rectum, or a megarectum secondary to previous anal obstruction, a higher than normal volume will be required both to activate the anorectal inhibitory reflex and to produce the appropriate sensation. It is not surprising that a number of children so endowed are able to withhold faeces for more than 10 days without suffering abdominal pain. It is also understandable why children who have been prone to severe constipation for many years are very unreliable in assessing the subtlety of rectal sensation and are victims of encopresis even when able to open their bowels regularly.

Problems with faecal expulsion

When the stool begins to descend, the anorectum should straighten. However, in a child who does not fully relax the voluntary muscles, or where the anus is rather anteriorly placed, the straightening may be incomplete. If the faecal mass is hard it may not be squeezed past these angulations by the rectal contractions above. This will lead to incomplete rectal emptying and further drying of the stools. A number of children can, by contracting their external sphincter and puboanalis sling, pull the descending stool back into the megarectum even though the internal sphincter has completely relaxed and the stool is seen clearly in the anal canal. They are highly motivated to avoid defaecation because of previous experience of the stool being forced through an incompletely relaxed anorectum by the rectal contractions at maximum rectal loading. Having experienced this pain, which is more intense the harder and larger the stool, the child decides to give up defaecation. If the anal pain is made worse by the development of an anal fissure, by an increase in parental anxiety or anger, or by the inappropriate use of suppositories or enemata, the stage is set for a long-standing problem.

It is clear from the relationship between the physiological events (rectal filling, distension, sensation, anal relaxation) and the psychological events (sensation perception, voluntary relaxation, learned defaecation, social responses) that when problems arise in this process a combined physical and psychological approach is required in every child irrespective of the initial cause.

References

1. Shapiro, O. (1948). Applied anatomy of infants and children: proctology. *Rev. Gastroent.* 15, 307–18.
2. Lawson, J. O. N. (1974). Pelvic anatomy. II. Anal canal and associated sphincters. *Ann. roy. Coll. Engl.* 54, 288–300.
3. Henry, M. M. (1988). Anorectal neuromuscular physiology. In *Anorectal surgery*, (ed. J. J. Decosse and I. P. Todd). Churchill Livingstone, Edinburgh.
4. Frenckner, B. and Ihre J. (1976). Influence of autonomic nerves on the internal anal sphincter in man. *Gut* 17, 306–12.

5. Lockhart, R. D., Hamilton, G. F., and Fyfe, F. W. (1969). *Anatomy of the human body*. Faber and Faber, London.
6. Hardcastle, J. D. and Parks, A. G. (1970). A study of anal incontinence and some principles of surgical treatment. *Proc. roy. Soc. Med* 63, 116–18.
7. Schuster, M. M. (1975). Progress in gastroenterology: the riddle of the sphincters. *Gastroenterology* 69, 249–62.
8. Phillips, S. E. and Edwards, D. A. W. (1965). Some aspects of anal continence and defaecation. *Gut* 6, 396–406.
9. Duthie, H. L. (1971). Progress report—anal continence. *Gut* 12, 844–52.
10. Lawson, J. O. N. (1974). Pelvic anatomy. *Ann. roy. Coll. Surg.* 54, 244–52, 288–300.
11. Parks, A. G., Porter, N. H., and Melzak, J. (1962). Experimental study of the reflex mechanism controlling muscles of the pelvic floor. *Dis. Col. Rect.* 5, 407–14.
12. Gaston, E. A. (1951). Physiological basis for preservation of faecal continence after resection of the rectum. *J. Am. med. Assoc.* 146, 1486–9.
13. Ottaviani, G. (1940). Histologische-anatomische untersuchungen uber die innervation des mesdarmes. *A. Mikroscop-Anat. Forsch.* 47, 151–82.
14. Denny-Brown, D. and Robertson, E. G. (1935). Investigation into the nervous control of defaecation. *Brain* 58, 256–310.
15. Templeton, R. D. and Lawson, H. (1931). Studies in the motor activity of the large intestine. 1. Normal motility in the dog by the tandem balloon method. *Am. J. Physiol.* 96, 667–76.
16. Connell, A. M. (1962). The motility of the pelvic colon. *Gut* 3, 342–8.
17. Code, C. E., Hightower, N. C., and Morlock, C. G. (1952). Motility of the alimentary canal in man. *Am. J. Med.* 13, 328–51.
18. Posey, E. L. and Bargan, J. A. (1951). Observations of normal and abnormal human intestinal motor function. *Am. J. med Sci.* 221, 10–20.
19. Grace, W. J., Wolf, S., and Wolff, H. (1951). *The human colon*. Harper & Row, New York.
20. Chaudhary, N. A. and Truelove, S. C. (1961). Human colonic motility: part III: Emotions. *Gastroenterology* 40, 27–36.

21. Gowers, W. R. (1877). The automatic action of the sphincter ani. *Proc. roy. Soc. Lond.* **26**, 77–84.
22. Porter, N. H. (1961). Megacolon: a physiological study. *Proc. roy. Soc. Med.* **54**, 1043–7.
23. Schuster, M. M., Hendrix, T. R. C., and Mendeloff, A. I. (1963). Internal anal sphincter response: manometric studies on its normal physiology, neural pathways and alteration in bowel disorders. *J. clin. Invest.* **42**, 196–207.
24. Lawson, J. O. N. and Nixon, H. H. (1967). Anal pressures in the diagnosis of Hirschsprung's disease. *J. ped. Surg.* **2**, 544–52.

3. Babies

DIETARY MANAGEMENT

Mothers feel their babies are frequently constipated and health visitors will be the first to vouch for this statement. Usually the constipation is of sudden onset and short duration with the baby having previously been well and passing normal bowel motions. There appears to be a lower incidence of this in breast-fed than in bottle-fed babies, although constipation in breast-fed babies is by no means rare. High osmolar bottle-feeds tend to cause dry stools and give rise to hard faeces, which predispose to the development of anal fissures and painful defaecation.[1] However, most modern cows milk formulae have osmolarity near to the physiological range. Typically, the history is of the baby becoming distressed intermittently with a red face and anxious look and seemingly in pain. Blood may have been noted in the stools or there may have been no proper passage of bowel motions in the previous 4–5 days. Usually the constipation is not long-standing enough to have lead to abdominal distension, although this may be seen. Defaecation is clearly very distressing not only to the child but also to the mother.

The most likely cause of the constipation is dietary. The history of fluid intake may be difficult to elicit if the child is breast-fed, but in bottle-fed babies this is easy. Constipation may have been noted after changing the type of bottle milk, or with the introduction of solids into the baby's diet.

The introduction of extra fluids, often in substantial quantities, either as water or fruit juices usually solves the problem. Occasionally, if the perianal area looks very raw with anal fissures some stool softener in small quantities (lactulose 2.5 ml b.d. (twice daily)) may be required initially, but this is usually not necessary. The constipation is unlikely to recur.

Constipation in babies can be summarized as follows.

(1) acute;

(2) short duration;

(3) dramatic improvement by increasing fluid intake;

(4) anal fissures, usually superficial, and rectal prolapse frequently seen.

OBSTRUCTED CONSTIPATION

Anal anomalies

These are as follows (see also Fig. 2):

(1) covered anus;

(2) anterior placed anus;

(3) ectopic anus;

(4) congenital anal stenosis;

(5) congenital anorectal stricture;

(6) imperforate anus;

(7) rectal atresia.

Anal anomalies can be divided into high or low anomalies depending on whether the anomaly is above or below the puborectalis sling (levator ani).[2] Low anomalies can be divided into those caused by:[3] (a) excessive fusion of the lateral genital folds resulting in the covered anus which may be found either at the normal anal site or when the anus is displaced forward; or (b) failure of the primitive cloaca to divide, accounting for most of the remainder of anal anomalies.

Minor anterior displacements of the anal canal and orifice are common[4] but it is uncertain whether these are generally of enough severity to cause distressful defaecation and constipation. However, severe anterior displacement of the

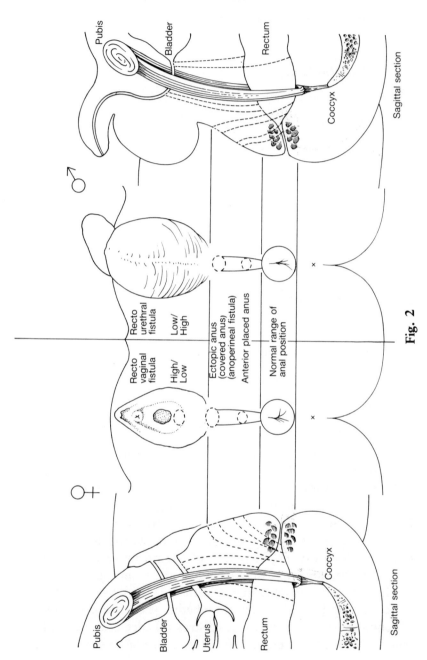

Fig. 2

Table 1. Anogenital index

	Boys	Girls
Newborn	0.58 ± 0.06	0.44 ± 0.05
4–18 months	0.56 ± 0.40	0.40 ± 0.06

anus is a well-recognized cause of constipation and this is more commonly seen in girls.[5] This anal malposition is easily overlooked at examination. In children normal values for the anal position on the perineum exist.[6] In boys the position is defined as the ratio of the anus–scrotum distance to the scrotum–coccyx distance and in girls the ratio is of the anus–fourchette distance to the fourchette–coccyx distance. This ratio is called the anal position index or anogenital index (see Table 1).

The ectopic anus in girls and the partially covered anus in boys are two examples of a low type of anal malformation, which is associated with an anterior anal displacement.[2]

Anal stenosis and anorectal strictures may be mild or severe. In many children with anal stenosis, the stenosis may resolve spontaneously by the end of the first year, presumably as the passing of stools acts as a dilator on its own. In other children one or two rectal digitations with a well-lubricated finger, in order to dilate the anal canal, is all that is required.[7] However, in some of the more severe cases the problem persists and can give rise to obstructive constipation with abdominal distension and an enlarged rectum.[8] These children need prompt surgical referral.

The imperforate anus is the most severe degree of anal obstruction. It can be divided into high, intermediate, and low types.

(a) High anal atresia—the bowel is clearly above the puborectal sling.

(b) Intermediate anal atresia—the termination of the bowel is at the level of the puborectal sling.

(c) Low anal atresia—the bowel is below and enwrapped by
     the puborectal sling; anus usually anteriorly placed on the
     perineum.

In low defects, anal fistula on the perineum in both sexes,
or rectovaginal fistulas in females, are not uncommon.[2]
Urinary fistulas are seen in high lesions. The types of atresias
may sometimes be distinguished by holding the baby upside
down for some minutes while allowing air to enter the most
distal part of the bowel.[9] With a little barium on the perineum
the thickness of the atresia can be defined. Occasionally, in
low atresias the obstruction is a thin diaphragm and this
requires minimal surgery. In high defects a colostomy is usually
required followed by corrective surgery 6–12 months later.

Most repairs of low imperforate anus results in good
continence but a significant proportion of those with high
defects are faecally incontinent. It should be remembered that
30 per cent of patients with imperforate anus have genito-
urinary problems, 10 per cent oesophageal atresia, and 7 per
cent have cardiac problems.

Associated congenital defects in the imperforate anus

These are: genito-urinary; oesophageal, cardiac, and vertebral.

Constipation secondary to other illness

The list on p. 42 illustrates some other illnesses which can give
rise to constipation.[10]

Hirschsprung's disease

Abnormalities of the myenteric nerve plexus will present as
constipation in babies. This is due to the failure of the
descending inhibitory impulses to relax the smooth muscle of
the bowel distally.

It is not surprising that the ganglion cells of the myenteric
plexus fail to reach the anus in some babies. The migration
of these parasympathetic neuroblasts starts from the cranio-
cervical neural crest, pass along vagal trunks, and reach the

cardia of the stomach by the sixth week of gestation. They continue to migrate caudally and, in spite of the rapid lengthening of the bowel, reach the end of the rectum by the twelfth week.[11] Auerbach's (myenteric) plexus is formed first and Meissner's (submucous) plexus is formed from this later.

The extrinsic parasympathetic innervation (from the vagal nucleus in the medulla for the right colon and the cell bodies in the sacral cord for the left colon and rectum) synapse with the ganglion cells of the myenteric plexus. If these pre-ganglionic fibres fail to find their ganglion cells they grow and branch dramatically, producing characteristic thickened nerve trunks in the area of the myenteric plexus and marked increase in acetylcholinesterase activity. This acetylcholinesterase activity can be used in the diagnosis of Hirschsprung's disease.[12,13] Since these frantic fibres grow even into the mucosa this allows the use of mucosal suction biopsies as a relatively safe form of biopsy in small babies and children.

The length of the aganglionic segment in Hirschsprung's disease is therefore variable. Total aganglionosis of the bowel occurs rarely (Zuelser–Wilson syndrome) and long-segment Hirschsprung's disease is less common than the short-segment type, approximately 10 per cent compared to 90 per cent respectively.[14] It is also clear from the variation in the age of presentation of the shorter segment disease that the segments appear to be of variable strength as well as length. This may reflect the balance of the parasympathetic, sympathetic, and other autonomic fibres in the aganglionic segment. When denervated smooth muscle tends to contract permanently (Cannon's Law),[15] so it is understandable that the aganglionic segment is narrow and obstructive. Historically, attention was paid to the enormously dilatated ganglionic proximal bowel and it was only Tittel who remarked on the paucity of ganglion cells in the narrow segment,[16] Hurst[17] who blamed Auerbach's plexus as having the abnormality leading to the anal sphincter achalasia, and then Whitehouse and Kernohan,[18] followed rapidly by Bodian, Stephens, and

Ward,[19] who proved the aganglionosis of the narrow segment in Hirschsprung's disease.

The *epidemiology* of Hirschsprung's disease may shed some light on the aetiology. It occurs in approximately 1 in 5000 live births. There is a risk of 3.6 per cent of another affected child being born to parents of a child with Hirschsprung's disease with boys being more at risk than girls. Familial cases with a much higher rate also occur. The marked male predominance in short-segment Hirschsprung's disease (8 : 1, male to female) reduces with the length of the colon affected, so that long-segment disease affecting the whole colon has an equal sex ratio.

There is a ten-fold increase in risk to children with trisomy 21. Of 1163 patients with Hirschsprung's disease, 24 had trisomy 21.[20] This tempts the formation of a unifying hypothesis to link both Hirschsprung's disease and Alzheimer's presenile dementia, both having demonstrable abnormalities of cholinergic neurones and known associations with trisomy 21. Apart from Down's syndrome, aganglionosis is related to very few syndromes compared to the structural anal anomalies. However, there is evidence that environmental factors may play an aetiological role, such as nutritional deficiencies, irradiation, rubella, and thalidomide.[21]

Clinical suspicion of Hirschsprung's disease

As described above there are many reasons for a baby to suffer from constipation. The diagnosis of Hirschsprung's disease is relatively straight-forward when the baby presents with acute lower intestinal obstruction soon after birth. Here, the surgeon's task is to distinguish between other causes such as meconium ileus of cystic fibrosis, ileus of septicaemia, lower bowel atresia, or volvulus. A barium enema will give the diagnosis in most cases presenting soon after birth. The difficulty arises when the segment is so short that the baby's early, more liquid, faeces can pass, and constipation occurring around weaning is the presenting feature. The shorter the segment the more likely it is that the child will present later in infancy (or later still if breast-fed). Here are some features which should increase the suspicion of Hirschsprung's disease in a constipated child.

- delay in passing meconium with or without abdominal distension;

- constipation starting from first week of life;

- vomiting;

- alternating constipation and diarrhoea;

- severe abdominal distension;

- failure to gain weight along expected centile;

- temporary improvement following rectal examination (this is often followed by an explosive passage of liquid faeces and gas);

- less overflow faecal soiling than expected with the degree of faecal loading (in older children);

Although Hirschsprung's disease is an uncommon cause of constipation, the risk of necrotizing enterocolitis makes the consideration of this diagnosis very important. An unprepared barium enema will show a short, narrow segment with a funnel-like transitional zone and a suction biopsy, with or without anorectal manometry, will usually confirm the diagnosis (see Chapter 8 on Investigations). The surgeon will then need to perform a relieving colostomy as an emergency in most cases.

The *ultra short-segment Hirschsprung's disease* variant tends to present later and elude diagnosis.[22] A barium enema will show a megarectum/megacolon only with no narrow or transitional segment. However, anorectal manometry will show failure of anal sphincter relaxation with rectal distension and the acetylcholinesterase activity of the rectal biopsy sample will be excessive. Internal anal sphincterotomy[23] will treat most of these cases effectively and provide deeper tissue to confirm the diagnosis histochemically. The above list of suspicious clinical features will be helpful with the ultra short-segment variant as well, but may be more subtle and merge with the features of idiopathic megarectum.

Colonic neuronal dysplasia
(neuronal intestinal dysplasia)

The absence of the ganglion cells of the myenteric plexus, as occurs in Hirschsprung's Disease, is only one abnormality of the so-called 'gut brain'. It is boasted by those interested in gut motility that there are more nerve cells in the gut than in the brain. The aganglionic segment in Hirschsprung's disease may be associated with a zone of colonic neuronal dysplasia—CND—(hyperganglionosis) with enlarged nerve trunks and excessive acetylcholinesterase activity.[24] There is also an association of CND with anorectal malformations.[25] It is, therefore, not surprising that some children have CND with neither Hirschsprung's disease nor malformations. These children present with constipation, sometimes poor feeding, and evidence of disordered colonic motility. They must be distinguished from children with chronic intestinal pseudo-obstruction (who often have failure to thrive and bladder problems with abnormal smooth muscle on histology).[26] Similarly, great care must be taken to exclude a very short-segment Hirschsprung's disease.

The difficulty of an exact histological diagnosis becomes even more problematic when there may be pressure from parents for a surgical solution to the child's distressing condition—even to the demand for colectomy. In some this is out of understandable desperation but in others it is a feature of 'Munchhausen by proxy'.

References

1. McCrae, W. M. (1984). *Textbook of paediatrics*, 3rd edn, (ed. J. O. Forfar and G. C. Arneil), p. 473. Churchill Livingstone, Edinburgh.

Obstructed constipation 25

2. Atwell, J. D. (1987). *Operative surgery and management*, 2nd edn, (ed. G. Keen), Wright, Bristol.
3. Nixon, H. H. (1984). Review of anorectal anomalies. *J. roy. Soc. Med. Suppl.* 3 77, 279–9.
4. Hendren, W. H. (1978). Constipation caused by anterior location of the anus and its surgical correction. *J. ped. Surg.* 13, 505–12.
5. Leape, L. L. and Ramenofsky, M. L. (1978). Anterior ectopic anus: a common cause of constipation in children. *J. ped. Surg.* 13, 627–30.
6. Reisner, S. H., Sivan, Y., Nitzan, M., and Merlob, P. (1984). Determination of anterior displacement of the anus in newborn infants and children. *Pediatrics* 73, 216–17.
7. Patton, E. F. and Hills, B. (1945). Proctological problems of the pediatrician. *J. Ped.* 27, 532–9.
8. Kiely, E. M., Chopra, R., and Corkery, J. J. (1979). Delayed diagnosis of congenital anal stenosis. *Arch. Dis. Childh.* 54, 68–70.
9. Filston, H. C. and Izant, R. (1978). *The surgical neonate. Evaluation and care.* Appleton–Century–Crofts, New York.
10. Ewerbeck, H. (1976). *Differential diagnosis in pediatrics.* Springer Verlag, New York.
11. Okamoto, E. and Ueda, T. (1967). Embryogenesis of intramural ganglia of the gut and its relation to Hirschsprung's disease. *J. ped. Surg.* 2, 437–43.
12. Meier-Ruge, W. (1968). Das megacolon, seine Diagnòse und Pathophysiologie. *Virchows. Arch. Abt. A* 344, 67–85.
13. Meier-Ruge, W. (1972). Hirschsprung's disease: aetiology, pathogenesis and diagnosis. *Curr. Top. Pathol.* 59, 131–79.
14. Wyllie, G. G. (1957). Treatment of Hirschsprung's disease by Swenson's operation. *Lancet* i, 850–5.
15. Bayliss, W. M. and Starling, E. H. (1901). The movements and innervation of the small intestine. *J. Physiol.* 26, 125–38.
16. Tittel, K. (1901). Uber eine angeborene Missbildung des Dietdarmes. *Wiener Klin. Woch.* 39, 904–7.
17. Hurst, A. (1934). Anal achalasia and megacolon. *Guys Hospital Report* 84, 317–50.
18. Whitehouse, F. R. and Kernohan, J. W. (1948). Myenteric plexus in congenital megacolon. *Arch. intern. Med.* 82, 75–111.

19. Bodian, M., Stephens, F. D., and Ward, B. C. H. (1949). Hirschsprung's disease and idiopathic megacolon. *Lancet* i, 6–11.
20. Passarge, E. (1967). The genetics of Hirschsprung's disease. Evidence for heterogenous etiology and a study of sixty-three families. *New Eng. J. Med.* **276**, 138–43.
21. Ehrenpreis, T. (1970). *Hirschsprung's disease*, pp. 47–9. Year Book Medical Publications, Chicago.
22. Clayden, G. S. and Lawson, J. O. N. (1976). Investigation and management of long standing chronic constipation in childhood. *Arch. Dis. Childh.* **51**, 918–23.
23. Bentley, J. F. R. C. (1966). Posterior excisional anorectal myotomy in management of chronic faecal accumulation. *Arch. Dis. Childh.* **41**, 144–7.
24. Puri, P., Lake, B. D., Nixon, H. H., Mishalamy, H., and Clareaux, A. E. (1977). Neuronal Colonic Dysplasia: an unusual association with Hirschsprung's disease. *J. ped. Surg.* **12**, 681–5.
25. Fadda, B., Meier, W. A., Meier-Ruge, W., Scharli, A., and Daum, R. (1983) Neuronale intestinale Dysplasie. Eine kritische 10-Jahres—Analyse Klinischer und Bioptischer Diagnose. *Z. Kinderchir.* **38**, 305–11.
26. Glassman, M., Spivak, W., Mininberg, D., and Madara, J., (1989). Chronic Idiopathic Intestinal Pseudo-obstruction: A commonly misdiagnosed disease in infants & children. *Pediatrics* **83**, 603–8.

4. Toddlers

THE ROLE OF DIET

The diet and bowel habits of infants and toddlers vary. Most one to four-year old children seem to eat a diet low in fibre. The onset of constipation may be related to an intercurrent illness with poor appetite and dry, hard stools. Initially, increasing the fluid intake as in babies may be helpful but usually the diet can be improved and items rich in fibre may be added (see Table 2).

Table 2. Dietary sources of fibre

1. Wholemeal bread and wholemeal flour.

2. Rye crispbread.

3. Some breakfast cereals (Bran flakes, Weetabix, Puffed and Shredded Wheat, porridge oats, muesli, Shreddies, Mini wheats).

4. Beans, peas, and lentils.

5. Nuts and dried fruit; such as dates, figs, currants, sultanas, raisins.

6. Brown rice and wholewheat pastas; such as macaroni and spaghetti.

7. Fresh fruit and vegetables; especially those eaten with their skins, e.g. unpeeled baked potatoes.

Bran may be added to the diet of the young child by spreading it over breakfast cereals for instance. However, too much fibre can be potentially harmful to the child's growth and general nutrition.[1] Presumably this is because fibre takes up considerable room in the stomach and may reduce the child's appetite for other food items.

Late presentation of obstructed constipation

Children with congenital anomalies of the anal canal or with Hirschsprung's disease and other neuronal disorders of the hind gut can present after the first two years of life with constipation. There may be gross faecal loading with severe abdominal distension and a megarectum. Severe anal stenosis may present in this way and most of the Hirschsprung's disease presenting at this stage is of the short-segment type.[2] With delay in diagnosis there is the risk of a toxic megacolon developing with life-threatening complications.

BEHAVIOUR DISTURBANCE ASSOCIATED WITH POT TRAINING

There is an enormous variation in the timing of continence training (pot training) between cultures. The Taira, a Japanese rural community, commence training at about 10 months[3] whereas the Nyansongo in Kenya start after the age of two years. It is of note that the age at which the child achieves continence appears to be similar, at around 2–3 years.

Many parents will notice that the gastrocolic reflex produces a stool after a feed is taken by young infants. Some babies are so reliable in this activity that the parents take the opportunity to catch the stool in a carefully placed pot after, or towards the end of, a feed. This may be successful for a while but in the second year of life the child gains more control and the apparent success breaks down. This may lead to great disappointment in the parents and an assumption that the child is either ill or naughty. This may then lead on to inappropriate medication or coercive methods to force the child to defaecate as regularly as the reflex produced previously. Some parents are misled by their parent's boasts of success with them at very young ages. Complicated regimes and remedies are advised by these smug grandparents and the child is treated instead of being observed. Most children will alter their behaviour as they perceive the contraction of the rectum. They may stand very still, look vacant or entranced, and blush slightly around their nasal folds and eyes. These early signs can be noticed by an attentive parent, allowing the child to be put on the pot with only seconds before a stool appears. The child and parent (the potting couple[4]) are then rewarded with a stool, framed in the pot in full glory. If this is praised honestly, the child will be keen to achieve further acclaim by repeating the activity each time the appropriate rectal sensation is perceived.

This ideal situation can be sabotaged by:

(1) The parent imposing the pot when the child is not ready to use it.

(2) The parent missing the subtle cues of imminent defaecation. (This is a possible link between the four times more common speech-delay noted in constipated children compared to other children—possibly the parent failing to pick up the child's cues because the parent is either absent or inattentive because ill, or busy, or unmotivated.)

(3) The parent greeting the arrival of the stool with horror or disgust.

(4) The child and parent becoming locked in a battle of wills.

(5) The child experiencing anal pain due to a hard stool or anal fissure.

(6) The child being unable to defaecate because of a too large stool.

(7) The child noting that there is a difference of opinion between parents/grandparents and becoming afraid of the stressed atmosphere associated with the use of the pot.

Management tactics

Problems could be prevented by avoiding the above factors. If the problem is established the pot should be put away for a few months and reintroduced when memories have faded. Coercive methods should be discouraged and rewards instituted. If the child is able to avoid defaecation, it may be necessary to alter the diet or add a stool softener to make constipation less likely in those prone to it. Most children will withhold for the time they are on the pot only to defaecate as they move away. Parents should be advised to react to this with patience as it is not as defiant a response as it appears.

Success with micturition usually predates that with defaecation and this can be used as part of the game to familiarize the child with the praise potential of the pot. This area of potential clash of wills will inevitably amplify any existing difficulty in family relationships. If the simple measures fail then a more detailed assessment of the family dynamics is necessary.

THE ROLE OF ANAL PAIN

Pain is a very powerful learning stimulus in early childhood. The exploring child very soon learns to associate certain activities with pain and so avoids potentially damaging experiences. At around the same developmental stage, the ability to control the previously automatic defaecation response begins. Sensations from the rectum begin to reach the child's consciousness. They appear to experiment in contracting the pelvic floor muscles and the external anal sphincter, long before real social continence is achieved. If they experience pain during defaecation they will contract the voluntary muscles in a reflex response to stop the pain in the same way as they would withdraw from touching a sharp or hot object. Unfortunately, the sudden contraction of the external sphincter is likely to grip onto the offending stool and lead to more pain and more focused fear.

If the stool is hard due to dietary fluid or fibre deficiency, or due to prolonged residence in the rectum, the pain will be intensified. The dragging effect of the stool on the mucosa of the anal canal, which has been gripped by the sphincter spasm, leads to the tearing down of the delicate anal folds. A fissure is easily formed in this way. In our prospective study of 146 severely chronically constipated children 75 per cent had a history of painful defaecation and 55 per cent had a history of passing blood during defaecation.

The toddlers will then react in two main ways. If they have a rectal capacity to allow it, they will give up defaecation. They may pass many days without opening their bowels and then spend one or two days in fear and agony until the critical volume of the rectum is reached and the then large, hard stool comes out, with further pain and confirmation that defaecation is worth avoiding at all costs. The other way they may react if they do not have a permissively large rectum, is to scream for a few hours before each stool is passed but without being able to withhold for long. They are less likely to pass very large or hard stools and even if they are afraid, they are likely to go as they fall asleep or awaken. The problem may be exaggerated by the response of desperate parents to the screaming. If this provokes anxiety in the parent, and especially if the parent converts this into anger, a major breakdown in the relationship and an increase in the child's fear will occur. If the child is unluckily taken to a doctor who prescribes a suppository or enema, the scene is set for major battles.

So, to summarize, whatever caused the original pain or anal soreness the child's reluctance to defaecate will be increased by:

● capacity of rectum before obligatory defaecation;

● hardness of the stool;

● sensitivity of the anal canal (± anal fissure);

● parents' response to the distressed child;

● inappropriate medical intervention.

Management tactics

Careful explanation might help the parents to defuse the situation, although attempts to persuade the child at this age will almost certainly fail. Stool softeners such as docusate (if residual stools are palpable per abdomen) or lactulose or methyl cellulose will help. In those children with a rectal capacity sufficient to allow many days withholding, a stimulant laxative such as senna will be necessary to ensure more regular defaecation. This will reduce the risk of the stool becoming harder and larger and will reduce the 'major event' nature of the final moment of defaecation. Once the child has learned this unfortunate response to the rectal sensation of imminent defaecation, it will take many months of the comfortable passage of stools to extinguish the fear. For this reason laxatives are likely to be necessary for the same period.

References

1. Zoppi, G., Gobio–Casali, L., Deganello, A., Astolfi, R., Saccomani, F., and Ceccheltin, M. (1982). Potential complications in the use of wheat bran for constipation in infancy. *J. ped. Gastroent. Nutr.* 1, 91–5.
2. Doig, C. M. (1984). Childhood constipation and late presenting Hirschsprung's disease. *J. roy. Soc. Med. Suppl. 3* 77, 305.
3. Whiting, B. B. (1963). *Six cultures. Studies in child rearing. Laboratory of human development.* John Wiley, New York.
4. Anthony, E. J. (1957). An experimental approach to the psychopathology of childhood: encopresis. *Brit. J. med. Psychol.* 30, 146–75.

5. Children

Here we present some descriptive data on children with chronic constipation seen over the last 10 years which is similar to other surveys on smaller numbers of children.[1,2] These data were collected with standardized questionnaires from 230 children and stored on computer for analysis.[3] The clinical features provide some confirmation of the model of the pathophysiology and the interaction between the physical and psychological factors.

CLINICAL FEATURES

There was a 2 : 1, male to female ratio and a bimodal frequency of the age of onset, with peaks soon after birth and around 2 years of age. This suggested a double population, one with early physical difficulties in defaecation and one with later difficulties precipitated by the strains of pot training.

The time interval between stools was recorded, where many children had delays of over two weeks between stools. A longer time interval between stools was noted in older children and those with noticeable psychological problems. Associated faecal incontinence occurred in 70 per cent of all the constipated children (nearly equally divided between continuous soilers and those whose soiling remitted after passing their delayed stool).

The suggestion that anal pain may play a major role in the development of chronic constipation is supported by the finding that 60 per cent were reported to pass hard stools, 45 per cent had a history of always passing massive stools (frequently requiring expert plumbing assistance to unblock the lavatory), and all but 14 per cent had passed massive stools at some stage. Painful defaecation was recorded in 74 per cent of the

constipated children, and blood noted in the stool by a parent
in 55 per cent.

The commonly held view that most constipation in childhood
is predominantly dietary is only partly supported by this study.
A 'good' appetite was reported in 37%, 'fair' in 15%, 'poor
if loaded' in 25%, 'poor' in 22%, and 'excessive' in 1%.

The children studied were, by their referral to a central clinic,
likely to be the more protracted cases; the parents recognized
abdominal distension in 61 per cent. Anxiety about defaecation
was very common and there was a clear history of pot or
lavatory refusal in 62 per cent.

The relationship with urinary problems is well recognized.
Many urologists are reluctant to attempt to manage bladder
problems until coexistent constipation is under reasonable
control. Enuresis occurring after 6 years of age was reported
in 13%, a history of urinary retention episodes in 16%, and
previously diagnosed urinary tract infections in 12% of the
constipated children studied.

There was a family history of constipation in 49 per cent
(mother 26%, father 13%, sibling 10%, maternal grandmother
11%, cousin 3%). Seven per cent of the mothers had taken
laxatives in pregnancy.

The average birth weight was 3.2 kg and average gestational
age 39.6 weeks. There was a history of neonatal intestinal
obstruction in 7% and feeding difficulties in 19%. Ribbon
stools in infancy were described in 13%.

All the children had had some previous treatment for
constipation at the time of referral; 67% senna, 63%
suppositories, 38% enemata, 33% in-patient treatments,
7% disimpactions under general anaesthetic, and 15% had
had, or were having, psychotherapy. Speech delay was reported
in 24% (compared to 7.2% in males and 4.4% in females in
the National Child Development Survey[4]). School or learning
problems occurred in 30% (children with mental subnormality
or other neurological illnesses were excluded from this survey).
The problems associated with soiling at school were not
included in this category. The high incidence of difficulties at

school could not be explained merely by a social class effect because there was a similar social class distribution to that of London and the south east of England, only 11 per cent were from single parent families, but 27 per cent of the families had a history of psychiatric disturbance. Attempts to define the emotional stability were approximated by: parental description of the child's behaviour as: normal 47%, sociable 14%, aggressive 13%, and shy 26%; and by the author, following the first consultation, as: normal 60%, very shy 21%, retarded 4%, aggressive 2%, immature 5%, anxious 5%, and depressed 2%.

On examination abdominal distension was present in 39 per cent and faecal masses palpable per abdomen in 67 per cent. This was graded according to the level of the upper border of the faecal mass as follows:

just palpable, 11%;

halfway to umbilicus, 14%;

level of umbilicus, 20%;

one third of distance from umbilicus to xiphisternum, 15%;

two thirds of distance from umbilicus to xiphisternum, 5%;

level of xiphisternum (usually associated with dyspnoea), 1%.

The length of time on stimulant laxatives was used as some guide to the severity of the condition and Table 3 shows the significant features which were associated with a shorter or longer treatment time (multivariant analysis was used to test the statistical significance).

It is possible to understand the features of constipation in childhood, such as those observed above, if the patho-physiology of the megarectum is considered. As described on page 12 (Chapter 2, physiology section), the greater than normal size rectum is more likely to become impacted with hard faeces than a normal size one. Figure 3 (page 58 in Chapter 7) demonstrates the vicious cycles which lead

Table 3. Summary of the factors influencing the length of treatment needed

Associated with shorter length of treatment	Associated with more protracted length of treatment
Onset around pot training	Early onset
No soiling	Continuous soiling
Older children with soiling	Young children with soiling
Marked psychiatric factors (N.B. receiving psychotherapy)	Long delays between defaecation
No obvious psychiatric factors	Possible/probable psychiatric factors (most not accepting or receiving psychotherapy)
Positive history of infantile colic	Social class V and unclassified
Aggressive behaviour (parents' description) in social class 1, 2, 3N	Aggressive behaviour and speech problems
Pot refusal	Father coercing child with marked psychiatric factors
Parental coercion	
No faecal collection on examination	Marked faecal collection on examination
Rapid, low-amplitude rhythmical activity, maximum during closing activity or early inflation (similar to enuretics)	Slow, high-amplitude rhythmical activity, maximum inflation (similar to Hirschsprung's Disease)
Therapeutic anal dilatation	No sensation during anorectal manometry.

to the distressing complications of overflow faecal incontinence, anal pain, and difficulty in defaecation.

THE PATHOPHYSIOLOGY
OF THE MEGARECTUM

A number of the presenting features of chronic constipation in children can be explained by considering a model of the disturbed physiology of that region of the body. The main features are:

- capacity of the rectum;

- sensation of urgency of defaecation;

- degree of anal inhibition in response to rectal distension;

- motivation to relax voluntary continence muscles;

- effectiveness of rectal propulsive action.

Capacity of the rectum

Although impossible to prove because of ethical considerations, the rectal capacity of children at different ages is likely to be distributed over a normal range; in a similar way to height, weight, and head circumference. The familial tendency to constipation could be explained by their having rectal capacities above the 90th centile. When endowed with a larger than average size rectum, the child inevitably requires more faecal loading to induce an urgent sensation to defaecate and to completely inhibit the internal anal sphincter smooth muscle activity. This child is also at a greater risk of the stool drying and hardening when accumulating in the rectum, which, like the rest of the colon, is still absorbing fluid. As obligatory defaecation occurs infrequently, this becomes an event of importance to the child and the family with expectation, anxiety, and the fear of pain from the hard, dry stool.

It is unproven whether the capacity of the rectum is significantly increased by persistent faecal loading, or whether this merely illustrates the original capacity of the rectum. The response of many children to therapeutic avoidance of chronic overloading of the rectum would favour the belief that the rectal capacity is, to some extent, plastic. However, evidence that children have a tendency to relapse even after many years of managing without constipation, together with the evidence of anorectal physiology,[5] supports the belief that they have permanently larger than average size rectums. The truth probably lies somewhere between these two views, with each child having a degree of both congenital and acquired causes of the large capacity. A number of children appear to function quite efficiently until they reach a particular degree of faecal loading, at which point they appear to decompensate rapidly. This may indicate that the rectum has become so enlarged that it cannot contract effectively (a kind of Starling's Law of the rectum!), or more likely that the retained faecal mass has become an impossible shape to pass through the anorectum or even the bony pelvic outlet (faeco-pelvic disproportion).

Sensation of urgency of defaecation

The sensation of a full rectum and the frequent feeling of the need to defaecate drives most individuals to search for a convenient place to relieve these unpleasant demands. During anorectal manometry it can be observed that the maximum sensation occurs during the rectal contraction seen in response to deliberate rectal distension (see page 77). In children with megarectum, this sensation occurs at volumes of rectal distension much greater than normal[2] and we found that those who experienced no sensation during the rectal distension stage of anorectal manometry were more likely to need longer laxative treatment than those where the sensation of the call to stool was experienced. So, as most of us find, the need to defaecate is at least annoyingly time-consuming and at worse frightening because of the risk of anal pain. If this is not rewarded by the pleasant relief of the cessation of rectal sensation, defaecation is likely to be postponed. This is another factor leading to delay in defaecation and apparent evidence to the child that all parental force or persuasion is unjust. This also seems to be one of the ways that stimulant laxatives may help. They appear to increase the discomfort of withholding faeces and therefore amplify the relief after the stool is passed.

   A number of children appear to have poor rectal sensation as a residual problem when the constipation element of their bowel problem has come under control. This leads to encopretic accidents even when the overflow soiling has ceased. Anorectal manometry demonstrates to them how their muscles are relaxing. They are sometimes able to perceive subtle sensations and learn to use these to avoid further problems (see biofeedback, page 54). It is debatable whether the apparent lack of urgent sensation is a result of local rectal sensory deficit or a more central block by their minds, protecting them from perceiving a reminder of the area in their bodies which has given them such bad experiences in the past.

Degree of anal inhibition in response to rectal distension

As described in the section on Hirschsprung's disease (page 20), the recto-anal reflex is very important in permitting effective defaecation. Children with non-Hirschsprung's megarectum do not relax the internal (involuntary) anal sphincter normally in response to rectal distension.[2,6] Even isolated strips from the internal anal sphincter of constipated children treated by internal anal sphincterotomy appear to have a contraction to acetylcholine *in vitro*, rather than the relaxation seen in adult control strips.[7] This may reflect the original obstructive cause of the megarectum or merely be a response to the smooth muscle hypertrophy of the anorectum. The inhibition of the internal anal sphincter is composed of two parts. The first is a rapid relaxation which inversely mirrors the rectal contraction wave. The second is a more sustained fall in pressure which drops further with each increment in rectal distension, until obligatory defaecation occurs. In the constipated child, the early partial relaxations are sufficient to allow the seepage of loose faecal matter to soil the underclothing. However, the failure or delay in complete relaxation obstructs the passage of the large, retained faecal mass. The rationale behind performing vigorous anal dilatations under general anaesthesia, or internal anal sphincterotomy, is to reduce the obstructive nature of the internal anal sphincter and allow the child to defaecate at a lower degree of rectal filling.

Motivation to relax the voluntary continence muscles

As explained in the section on continence (page 8) defaecation occurs when the continence muscles are deliberately relaxed. This reflex action gradually comes under conscious control as the child develops. If defaecation is rewarded by pain, shame, or disgust, this conditioning is perverted. Instead of relaxing the external sphincter and the puboanalis, the child contracts these and pulls the stool back from the sensitive, upper anal canal zone. Many parents will report seeing the stool beginning to emerge through the relaxed internal sphincter, only to disappear back into the rectum by a sudden contraction of the anus. Fortunately, the external sphincter fatigues after 30 seconds in children and so, if the rectum continues to contract and the internal sphincter is fully inhibited defaecation becomes obligatory however much the child protests. Clearly, if the child has a large capacity rectum, a partially inhibiting internal anal sphincter, and a hard, rounded stool, then deliberate attempts to withhold are reinforced. The same child will also have more reason, from memories of anal pain, to avoid defaecation. The apparent attempts of young children to defaecate (the episodes of straining graphically reported by the parents) are usually caused by the child using every available muscle to avoid defaecation. The child usually strains with legs straight and back arched when trying to put off the dreaded moment.

Effectiveness of rectal propulsive action

This is difficult to measure accurately but may vary between children with chronic constipation at different degrees of faecal loading. There has been debate as to whether a rectosigmoid sphincter exists and whether incompetence of this would lead to retrograde faecal movement during rectal contraction. One myth should be laid to rest, however, and that is the concept of rectal inertia in children. However large the rectum is, it still contracts actively and churns the retained stool into its unstreamlined ball shape. The frustrated rectal waves, with the partial internal anal sphincter relaxation, lead to the continuous faecal soiling so characteristic of the chronically constipated child.

If the rectal wall is observed during some forms of surgery in severe cases, or at autopsy in children who have died as a result of unrelated trauma, it is seen to be grossly hypertrophied. This is an important concept in the planning of therapeutic intervention. The gross hypertrophy of the anorectum in severely affected children would indicate that stimulant laxatives alone are unlikely to be effective. The obstructive nature of the anus must be confronted. The obstructing faecal mass must be removed. The rectum can normally propel its contents when sufficiently soft and malleable through a reasonably relaxed anal canal. The stimulant laxatives can then improve the chances of defaecation by improving the mass delivery to the rectum, thus generating a sudden rectal filling, rectal contraction, rectal sensation, anal canal inhibition, complete emptying, and more rewarding sense of relief.

CONSTIPATION AND ABDOMINAL PAIN

Abdominal pain is a presenting complaint in approximately 7 per cent of constipated children.[1] Conversely constipation was seen in 5 per cent of school children with abdominal pain.[8] Girls are more likely to present in this manner, particularly in the age range 6–10 years. The pain is often sudden and colicky in nature and, characteristically, the patient may not have had proper bowel motions for a considerable period of time. The child may be unable to have bowel motions and is very distressed. Examination often reveals a hard and faecally loaded abdomen. Evacuation of the bowel will break the vicious circle and occasionally this may require hospital admission. Such episodes can occur every few weeks. These patients' diet is usually very poor in fibre.

Many children give a history of milder abdominal discomfort or pain which is immediately relieved by spontaneous defaecation. This causes minimal distress and is characteristically seen in younger children.

Abdominal pain is associated with a good prognosis.[1]

Abdominal pain in constipation is associated with:

(1) girls;

(2) good prognosis;

(3) faecal loading;

(4) diet poor in fibre.

CONSTIPATION SECONDARY TO OTHER ILLNESS

The following list illustrates some other illnesses which give rise to constipation.

1. Hypothyroidism, should be diagnosed as prolonged jaundice, umbilical hernia, hypothermia, hypotonia, etc.

2. Renal tubular acidosis, particularly of the proximal tubular type, with hypercalcaemia and failure to thrive.

3. Hypercalcaemia in hyperparathyroidism and hypervitaminosis-D.

4. Hypokalaemia secondary to diarrhoeal illness.

5. Neurological/severe physical handicap.

6. Milk protein allergy, this usually presents as loose stools/diarrhoea.

7. Coeliac disease.

8. Pyloric stenosis.

9. Lead poisoning.

10. Any intercurrent illness with poor fluid intake and immobility.
11. Cystic fibrosis.
12. Spinal tumours.
13. Skin diseases, epidermolysis bullosa[9].

References

1. Abrahamian, F. P. and Lloyd-Still, J. D. (1984). Chronic constipation in childhood: a longitudinal study of 186 patients. *J. ped. Gastroent. Nutr.* 3, 460–7.
2. Loening-Baucke, V. A. (1989). Factors determining outcome in children with chronic constipation and faecal soiling. *Gut* 30, 999–1006.
3. Clayden, G. S. (1981). *Chronic constipation in childhood.* MD Thesis, University of London.
4. Davie, R., Butler, N., and Goldstein, H. (1972). *From birth to seven. The second report of the National Child Development Study.* Longman, London.
5. Loening-Baucke, V. A. (1984). Abnormal rectoanal function in children recovered from chronic constipation and encopresis. *Gastroenterology* 87, 1299–1304.
6. Clayden, G. S. (1988). Is constipation in childhood a neuro-developmental abnormality. *Disorders of gastrointestinal motility*, (ed. P. J. Milla). John Wiley, Chichester.
7. Paskins, J., Clayden, G. S., and Lawson, J. O. N. (1982). Pharmacological response of some isolated internal anal sphincter strips from chronically constipated children. *Scand. J. Gastroent.* 17, 155–6.
8. Apley, J. (1975). *The child with abdominal pains*, 2nd edn. Blackwell Scientific Publications, Oxford.
9. Clayden, G. S. (1990). Dysphagia and constipation in Epidermolysis bullosa. *Epidermolysis Bullosa*, (ed. G. C. Priestley, M. J. Tidman, J. B. Weiss, and R. A. J. Eady). D.E.B.R.A., Crowthorne.

6. Children with special needs

CONSTIPATION AND GLOBAL DEVELOPMENTAL DELAY

Children with global developmental delay seem to be prone to developing constipation. There are a number of potential causes, apart from their neurological and intellectual handicap. This could be poor fluid intake, vomiting, diet poor in roughage and fibre, decreased mobility due to delayed walking, etc. Some of the children have constipation, with the retaining of hard faeces, palpable abdominally, and difficult defaecation of small pellets of stool, while others have severe faecal incontinence with frequent soiling accidents. Due to developmental delay toilet training is difficult and many children never achieve full toilet training. It can also be hard to decide what part behavioural factors may play in the persistence of bowel symptoms in some of these children.

Management

1. If the child is constipated proceed as follows:

    ● increase fluid intake;

    ● give a diet rich in fibre;

    ● encourage mobility;

    ● consider a stool softener/osmotic agent (lactulose);

    ● and/or a stimulating agent (Senna);

● administer the occasional suppository (glycerine) if distressed;

● establish, if possible, a regular toiletting routine;

——→ improvement.

If no improvement consider anorectal manometry and anal dilatation.

2. If the child is soiling and is also constipated proceed as above.

● if no evidence of severe faecal loading is detected consider regular toiletting ± suppositories, and regular/occasional manual evacuation ± stool softener

——→ situation improves.

● if no improvement consider anorectal manometry, treat as a constipated child if anal tone is high, continue as before if anal tone is low.

CEREBRAL PALSY AND BOWEL PROBLEMS

The features of bowel problems in cerebral palsy are as follows:

constipation ≫ faecal incontinence

defaecation distress/difficulties occasionally present

While some children with cerebral palsy are prone to constipation, and a minority have problems with faecal incontinence, it seems that most of these children do not have any major problems with their bowels. As in children with global developmental delay, the cause of constipation may have many factors. There is no evidence of a specific type of brain lesion in cerebral palsy giving rise to constipation but it has been postulated that supraspinal control of colonic and anorectal motility is located in the pons.[1] Immobility is a predisposing factor and inco-ordination of muscles and increased striated muscle tone may cause secondary skeletal deformities, such as scoliosis and kyphosis, which render abdominal and pelvic muscles almost useless during defaecation. It is not surprising, therefore, that some patients experience considerable distress and difficulties with defaecation. This is presumably due to spasticity of the pelvic floor and lack of synchrony between the internal and external anal sphincters. The spastic pelvic floor may affect the puborectalis muscle sling, which forms the anorectal angle, in such a way that the passage of stool through the anal canal becomes difficult. This inability to evacuate the anorectum and distal bowel leads to retention and faecal overflow.

Preliminary evidence[2] suggests that in the first cm of the anal canal the resting tone is lower than normal, while in the second and third cm the tone is unchanged. This suggests that the tone of the internal sphincter is unaffected while that of its striated counterpart is reduced. This seems to indicate that in cerebral palsy the bowel smooth muscles of the anorectum are not severely affected as a rule and that, unless the pelvic spasticity is severe, the cause of constipation is related to diet and fluids. Feeding children with cerebral palsy can be difficult, particularly during the first few years of life when vomiting and regurgitation are commonly present, and at this time constipation is often found. When older, the children often feed better and the bowel control improves. However, in cerebral palsy there is no general rule and constipation can start later in childhood as well. Difficulties with chewing calls for liquidizing the food and this may render the food poor in fibre.

Institutions who look after children with cerebral palsy often add fibre to the childrens' breakfast cereals and this, with an otherwise healthy diet rich in fibre and with sufficient fluid intake, appears to keep constipation at bay in most cases.

Constipation and cerebral palsy: potential causes

1. Central nervous system damage? Lesion in pons?
2. Poor mobility.

3. Skeletal deformity with weak abdominal muscles.

4. Pelvic floor spasticity/weakness.

5. Poor intellect?

6. Poor fluid intake.) due to vomiting, regurgitation,
7. Poor diet/fibre intake) inability to chew or swallow

Management

● increase fluids

● give diet rich in fibre

⟶ improvement.

● if no improvement consider stool softener (lactulose)/bulking agent (methyl cellulose) ± stimulating agent (senna)

⟶ improvement.

● if no improvement consider anorectal manometry.
if high/normal anal tone consider anal dilatation.
if low anal tone start regular toiletting ± suppositories (glycerine).

SPINAL LESIONS AND THE NEUROGENIC BOWEL

Constipation and faecal incontinence are common in children with spinal lesions, such as transection of the cord, meningomyelocele, or tethering of the cord. In meningomyelocele, faecal incontinence of varying degrees is seen in over 90 per cent of patients.[3] In adolescence and young adulthood this leads to low self esteem, depression, and other psychological problems.[4] Adult patients with paraplegia have normal anal sphincter tone[5] in contrast to that found in meningomyelocele.[5]

In patients with simple cord transection both constipation and faecal incontinence are found. In meningomyelocele the clinical picture may be less clear, since the spinal lesion can be patchy and asymmetric. It has been found that unilateral spinal defects may have no effect on anal tone.[6] Therefore, the relationship between the spinal defect in meningomyelocele and the level of bowel control is sometimes unclear. In meningomyelocele, hydrocephalus is present commonly and the effect this may have on the intestinal and anorectal function further complicates the clinical picture. In meningomyelocele the majority of patients have little, if any, rectal sensation and are, therefore unaware when the bowel needs emptying. They are unable to squeeze with the external anal sphincter due to paralysis of the pelvic floor and are thus unable to retain faeces in the anal canal/rectum for any length of time. The combination of these factors often causes severe faecal incontinence.

We divide patients into those with high and those with low spinal lesions and this will sometimes explain the different degree of bowel control seen in these children.

High lesions ($\geqslant$ L 2). These patients are generally less mobile than those with low lesions. The spinal deformity can be extensive, with extreme short stature, limb contractures, etc. The anal pressure appears, on average, to be lower in these patients than in those with low lesions. Slow intestinal transit may lead to stasis of a large volume of faeces, which by the time they have been slowly propelled into the distal large intestine and rectum are suddenly expelled as a result of the anorectal inhibitory reflex without any previous warning. The striated external anal sphincter and pelvic floor muscles are incapable of temporarily withholding the stool.

Low lesions ($\leqslant$ L 3). Some of the children can walk; usually those with sacral lesions. Anal pressure is usually higher than in those with high lesions. Those with very low lesions (S 2–3) may have rectal sensation and are able to squeeze with the external sphincter to some extent and retain faeces in the rectum. However, some patients with low lesions (lumbo–sacral area) appear to have extremely low anal pressure, even lower than that seen in patients with high lesions, with no rectal sensation and no capacity to squeeze or contract the external sphincter/pelvic floor muscles. These patients suffer from severe faecal incontinence, often made worse by limited mobility. No correlation has been found between the extent of limb paralysis and bowel control, or between bladder and bowel control in meningomyelocele.[7]

We have found that the rectum in meningomyelocele seems less active during distension than in normal or constipated children. Whether this is the effect of long-standing faecal loading, or the effect of the primary neural lesion, is uncertain.

It seems that patients with low lesions use laxatives less than those with high lesions, suggesting that retention of faeces is greater in those with higher lesions.

Stroking the perianal skin or anocutaneous junction with an orange stick normally elicits the anocutaneous reflex with contraction of the external sphincter. It has been felt that this reflex is present or strong in those patients with high spinal cord damage whilst absent in those with low spinal cord damage, where the reflex arc has been directly interfered with and damaged by the spinal defect. The presence of this reflex has been used to plan bowel management.[8] Patients with the reflex present are said to empty the rectum by reflex when it is stimulated, i.e. by a suppository or with a finger. Patients without the reflex are said to require manual evacuation of faeces, enemata, etc. to empty the rectum since it is inactive and does not respond to stimulation. However, due to the patchiness of the spinal lesion in meningomyelocele we have found that the reflex may be absent when one would expect to find it and vice versa, suggesting that one cannot rely only on the reflex as a guide to management.

Meningomyelocele: findings on anorectal manometry[9]

● Anal pressure low in first cm of anal canal.

● Anal pressure variable in second and third cm of anal canal.

- Rhythmical anal activity—featureless or surprisingly active.
- Only a few patients can squeeze/contract with external sphincter.
- Defaecation of rectal balloon easy in most patients.
- Rectal sensation absent in all with high lesions and most of those with low lesions.
- Rectal activity during distension is decreased.

Meningomyelocele: nature of spinal lesions

Patients with high spinal lesions:

- Retention of faeces and constipation, leading to overflow incontinence.
- Oral laxatives commonly used.

Patients with low spinal lesions:

- Frequent accidents of faecal incontinence due to sphincter weakness rather than faecal retention.
- Oral laxatives often badly tolerated and may increase faecal incontinence.

Bowel management: assessment

A. History

What is the bowel pattern?

Is it mainly incontinence? How often? How severe?

Is it mainly constipation?

Are both considered to be present and is incontinence due to overflow?

What is the current therapy/management?

B. Examination

Assess intelligence and psychological state.

Check for presence of hydrocephalus—is it arrested?

What is the nature of the spinal/skeletal deformity?

What is the degree of mobility?

Is the anocutaneous reflex present?

Carry out abdominal and rectal examination for faecal masses.

C. *Investigations (if indicated)*

Consider anorectal manometry and assess the anal resting tone, rectal sensation, ability to squeeze, ability to defaecate, and the nature of the manometry trace, i.e. whether it is 'flat' or 'active'.

Management

1. *Toilet routine and physical assistance*

Establishing a regular toiletting routine is very important. The earlier this can be done the better. Young children should be taught to strain when they are old enough to understand what is meant. This can be done by asking them to blow into a balloon while defaecating or, if older, to hold their breath while bearing down. Since anal tone is generally reduced in these disorders, straining with sufficient intra-abdominal pressure generated may empty the distal bowel surprisingly effectively. Initially, it is acceptable that the toiletting takes place lying down, in the left or the right lateral position, on a bed or somewhere suitable, and that the bowel is evacuated into a nappy. As the children get older one should try to transfer the procedure to a sitting position if this is at all possible. A regular routine should be established where the patient empties their bowels into the toilet or potty a few times every day, or at least attempts to do so. The timing of this should be after all main meals, i.e. breakfast, lunch, and dinner, and the patient should sit on the toilet/potty for approximately 10 minutes each time. Linking these sessions to the meals is important so that advantage can be taken of the gastrocolic reflex, which is rapid in young children. It is therefore important that this type of programme is started early in childhood, i.e. from 2–3 years of age. Sometimes bowel evacuation is incomplete after 10 minutes and the patient may have to try again 20–30 minutes later in order to avoid a soiling accident. However, tough toiletting programmes such as this are time consuming and may not be practical for many children, in particular those who are at school, etc. Each child's bowel programme intensity should be realistically tailored to their needs and acceptance.

Manual evacuation of faeces may have to be carried out initially when a toiletting programme is beginning. This is often done in small or young children. If the toiletting is successful manual removal of faeces should only be done as a supplement at the end of toiletting if it is felt that the bowel has not completely emptied. With time one would hope that such invasive manoeuvres would only be necessary occasionally. In some patients a finger in the rectum or anus, rather than a full manual evacuation, is required to stimulate a bowel action and this may be done after an unsuccessful straining/defaecation session.

2. Diet

A high fibre diet is advisable in those children who have high spinal lesions and where faecal retention is the major characteristic. In some children with low spinal lesions, where anal tone is very low and severe faecal incontinence is present a high fibre diet may exacerbate the incontinence.[10] This is presumably due to a fibre-induced shortened gastrointestinal transit time. Therefore, some have even advocated a low-residue diet for those patients whose faecal incontinence is gross and deteriorates with the introduction of fibre.

3. Oral fluids

Sufficient fluid intake is important for keeping the stools relatively moist and this is particularly important in young children.

4. Suppositories or microenemata

These may be useful where regular toiletting is not sufficient to keep patients clean. Patients with a positive anocutaneous reflex, and/or anal pressures which are not excessively low on manometry, may benefit from this. Glycerine or bisacodyl suppositories introduced after an unsuccessful defaecation attempt may stimulate a rectal contraction and empty the distal bowel. If patients are clinically loaded and emptying is required within a short period of time microenemata can be used.

In patients with severely reduced anal tone the effect of anal therapy may be low as the medication tends to leak out from the anus again, particularly if the patient is sitting upright. These medications should be administered in the lateral, lying position.

5. Oral medication

In patients with high spinal lesions bulk-forming agents (methyl cellulose, ispaghula husk, etc.) are useful to keep the stools formed. Softening agents (lactulose, dioctyl sodium sulphosuccinate, etc.) are useful if the stools are dry or hard. Stimulating agents (senna, bisacodyl) can be useful in patients with chronic faecal loading. The timing of maximal action of senna is difficult to predict (between 12–24 hours) and administering it is an exercise of trial and error.

In those with low lesions, bulking agents are useful as these patients often seem to have pellet-like stools which leak out from the anus when least expected. Keeping the stools formed so that they may be felt and made easier to pass would seem logical. Stimulant laxatives in low dosages given either regularly or occasionally can be helpful. It should be remembered, however, that over zealous laxative therapy, even in small dosages, may lead to diarrhoea or loose stools in these children.

In a few patients with low lesions, who have very low anal tone on manometry and who suffer severe faecal incontinence, it may be worth trying anti-stimulant drugs, such as codein phosphate, in order to reduce the constant leak or flow of faecal material and pellets of stool from the rectum.

6. Biofeedback

Biofeedback has been used to treat faecal incontinence in children with cord lesions.[11,12] It involves teaching patients to respond to a certain stimulus (i.e. rectal stimulation or sensation) by contracting the external sphincter/pelvic floor muscles and thereby increasing the anal tone. Repeated sessions, where this is taught on a weekly or twice weekly basis for 2–3 months, have been reported to increase anal tone in some patients and reduce faecal incontinence. The object is to be able to recognize signals or sensations indicating that a bowel action is imminent and so enable patients to withhold stool in the rectum long enough for later evacuation at will, into the toilet or potty.

This treatment has been carried out with anorectal manometry equipment where the inflated rectal balloon stimulates the rectum and the anal sphincter tone and trace can be observed directly on a computer monitor, thus relaying information back to the patient. By either seeing the anorectal inhibitory reflex on the monitor screen or by feeling some induced rectal or abdominal stimulation the patient should be able to recognize when a squeeze or a contraction of the anus is appropriate. Gradually, all such visual, or informed, feedback is reduced and finally the patient should be able to carry out the desired manoeuvres without being told when the rectum is distended or being able to visualize it on the monitor screen.

In meningomyelocele, generally, it seems that this therapy is no more successful than a good behaviour-modification programme such as regular toiletting.[13] However, biofeedback may be appropriate for those children who are strongly motivated, with good intelligence, and have low spinal lesions with some rectal sensation.

References

1. Weber, J., Denis, Ph., Mihout, B., *et al.* (1985). Effect of brain stem lesion on colonic and anorectal motility. A study of three patients. *Dig. Dis. Scien.* 30, 419–25.
2. Agnarsson, U., Gordon, C., McCarthy, G., Evans, N., and Clayden, G. S. (1989). Anorectal function in children with severe cerebral palsy. *Gut* 30, A1474.
3. Loening-Baucke, V. A., Desch, L., and Wolraich, M. (1988). Biofeedback training for patients with myelomeningocele and fecal incontinence. *Dev. Med. child. Neurol.* 30, 78–90.
4. Riveille, C. (1962). Problems psychologiques dans le spina bifida paralytique. *Ann. med. Psychiatr.* 125, 5.
5. Meunier P. and Mollard, P. (1977). Control of the internal anal sphincter (manometric study with human subjects). *Pflügers Arch. ges. Physiol.* 370, 233–9.
6. Gunterberg, B., Kewenter, J., Petersen, I., and Stener, B. (1976). Anorectal function after major resections of the sacrum with bilateral or unilateral sacrifice of sacral nerves. *Br. J. Surg.* 63, 546–54.
7. Scobie, W. G., Eckstein, H. B., and Long, W. J. (1970). Bowel function in myelomeningocele. *Dev. Med. child Neurol. Suppl.* 22, 12, 150–6.
8. Rickwood, A. M. K. (1984). Bowel management for patients with spina bifida. *Link* (the ASBAH magazine) November/December, 6.
9. Agnarsson, U., Gordon, C., McCarthy, G., Evans, N., and Clayden, G. S. (1989). Anorectal function in children and adolescents with spina bifida. *Gut* 30, A715.
10. Shurtleff, D. B. (1980). Myelodysplasia: management and treatment. In *Current problems in pediatrics*, Vol. 10, no. 3. Year Book Medical Publishers, Chicago.
11. Wald, A. (1983). Biofeedback for neurogenic fecal incontinence: rectal sensation is a determinant of outcome. *J. ped. Gastroent. Nutr.* 2, 302–6.
12. Whitehead, W. E., Parker, L. H., Masek, B. J., Catalder, M. F., and Freeman, J. M. (1981). Biofeedback treatment of fecal incontinence in patients with myelomeningocele. *Dev. Med. child. Neurol.* 23, 313–22.

13. Whitehead, W. E., Parker, L., Bosmajian, L., *et al.* (1986). Treatment of fecal incontinence in children with spina bifida: comparison of biofeedback and behaviour modification. *Arch. phys. med. Rehabil.* **67**, 218–24.

7. The management of constipation

MANAGEMENT OF THE CHILD WITH CONSTIPATION

The main complaints from the children and their parents are that the delays in defaecation lead to overflow faecal incontinence and/or pain on defaecation. The other symptoms related to chronic faecal retention are listed in the clinical features section (p. 33) but the change in the child's personality, appetite, and energy levels with increasing faecal loading add to the distress caused by soiling and anal discomfort. The secrecy surrounding these particularly embarrassing conditions leads the families to believe that they are the only ones to be suffering from this. The nature of the symptoms, with the association with uncleanliness or neglect, make it unlikely that either the child or the parent will discuss the stress they are experiencing with their friends. In the professional management of these problems it is essential to demystify by explaining the physiological basis and to exonerate by tactfully listing the emotional and behavioural responses that many families show when living through these difficult times.

It is much easier to explain treatment regimes if the child and family share a conceptual model of the interaction of the factors causing the chronic problem. Figure 3 shows one way in which the various factors interact and it can be helpful with some families to use this diagram and annotate it to match the balance of factors for the individual child. Explanation is so essential that some form of written information should be given. For this reason the booklet which is available to our patients and families is shown in the Appendix and is presented in a form which allows easy photocopying. The other advantage of carefully explaining the condition is that

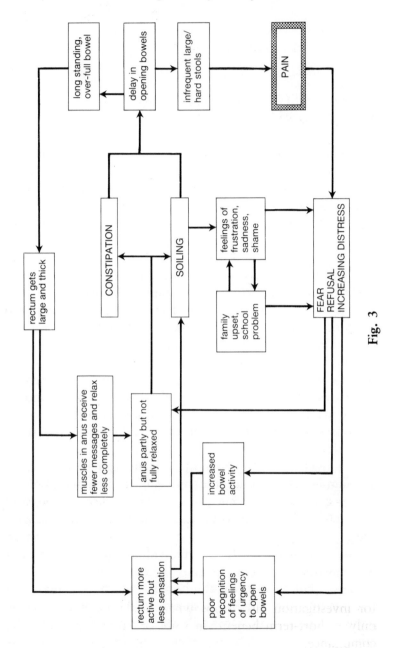

Fig. 3

areas of uncertainty arise which indicate the need for further investigation. Similarly, irrational treatments can be avoided by sharing a clear idea of the objective of the treatment prescribed.

Investigation

Details of investigation methods are given in Chapter 8 (page 70), but it may be helpful to consider when they should be carried out in relation to the ways in which the child may present. If the child is thriving, eating normally, and has no symptoms beyond the anorectum, then no investigations are necessary. The younger the child, the more distended, with the presence of vomiting, failure to thrive, and the relative lack of soiling, then the more suspicion there should be of an ultra short-segment Hirschsprung's disease (see page 23). At the other end of the scale, if a soiling child appears to have no evidence of faecal retention an abdominal X-ray may demonstrate faecal retention which was impalpable on abdominal examination. Persistence of symptoms, difficulty in explanation or reassurance, and unusual response to treatment are often indications that further investigation is needed, which might include barium enema, anorectal manometry, or rectal biopsy. These more invasive investigations should be avoided unless there are definite suspicions of Hirschsprung's disease or its variants, and should never be requested out of pure desperation or in response to parental pressure to 'do something'. In the older child, anorectal manometry might be useful in helping the child to link the physiological changes seen on the computer screen with their sensations. However, many children are alienated from rectal procedures at this stage, making any attempt at this form of biofeedback impossible. The threshold for investigation also drops when treatment regimes have only a short-term benefit, in spite of high motivation and compliance.

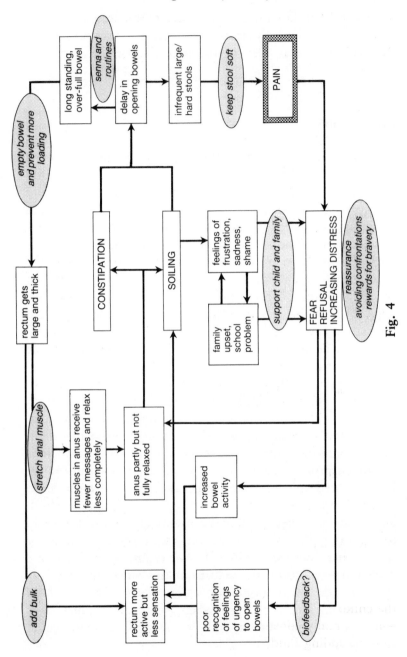

Fig. 4

Treatment

Treatment must be tailored to the individual child's needs and, as can be seen from the annotated diagram (Fig. 4), it should be possible to define the objective of each method in unravelling the vicious cycles. In this process, it is salutary to include the likely complications: this reduces the risk of unexpected failure.

The basic plan should be to:

- explain the problem fully;

- use the minimum therapeutic input;

- ensure complete evacuation of retained stools (see pages 66, 68);

- maintain regularity of bowel movement (see page 66);

- establish effective toiletting routines (see page 29 also);

- monitor progress (charts, consultations—personal and telephone);

- support child and family through the difficult times (see page 87);

- establish information network to ensure the above management.

The figure illustrates how these features may operate on the factors leading to the child's bowel problem.

MANAGEMENT ALGORITHM

This abbreviated management scheme summarizes the manoeuvres which are available, but the individual child must be treated with a tailored plan as described above.

After a full discussion with parents and examination of the child:
—if it is really constipation (delay and distress)
    —try adding fluid, fibre, lactulose

—if this fails
  AND
    the younger the infant
  OR
    the stronger the history of neonatal obstruction
                                 vomiting
                                 abdominal distension
                                 failure to thrive
                                 alternating diarrhoea

  THEN
      investigate as in-patient—observation by nurse
                                 calcium, TSH
                                   unprepared barium enema
                                 rectal biopsy ±
                                   anorectal manometry
(depending on severity of history and response to simpler
measures)

  OTHERWISE:
  —if hard faeces palpable per abdomen; use docusate
  —when no faeces palpable per abdomen; use lactulose
      or cologel
      —if fails, or delays more than three days between stools;
          add senna
  —when abdominally palpable faeces persist after docusate
      —if massive, or child acutely distressed; manual evacu-
          ation under general anaesthetic (G/A)
      —if moderate and child co-operative or deeply sedated;
          enema
      —if mild, try picosulphate

  THEN:
  —establish defaecation routine with senna, softener ±
      picosulphate, + attention to toileting routines and
      medicine compliance

—if fails to establish new routine, check causative factors:
  —if reluctance to use lavatory / pot involve psychologist /
   nurse
  —if frequent relapse or failure to improve soiling, check:
     —compliance with treatment and routines
     —effectiveness of evacuation (abdominal X-ray)
     —severity of megarectum; rectal biopsy
                             (anorectal manometry)
                             (barium enema)
—consider anal dilatation under G / A
—consider internal anal sphincterotomy in those temporarily responding to anal dilatation

(Any escalation of investigations and physical treatments must be balanced with psychological assessments and vice versa. Therefore, in-patient observation often indicated.)

DETAILS OF TREATMENTS

Dietary fibre

Many children can avoid constipation by increasing their intake of dietary fibre. A small change to increase fruit and sources of green fibre is likely to be of more benefit than attempting to add large volumes of bran. In children who have poor appetites or where eating is particularly difficult (e.g. epidermolysis bullosa) the volume of high fibre and low calorie intake may make the failure to thrive worse. When there are difficulties in achieving a high fibre diet bulking laxatives are helpful.

Bulk laxatives

These are thought to work by trapping water in the stool and by producing a larger but softer stool to aid the passage through the bowel. These can be helpful when a child is withholding faeces and suffering as a result of the stool becoming dry and hard. In those children with a degree of megarectum the larger volume entering the rectum from above is more likely to activate the appropriate recto-anal reflexes and maximize sensation. The stool frequency is improved and the fear lessened. Mild cases may respond to bulk laxatives alone but many will need a course of stimulant laxative for a period, although it is helpful to continue the bulk laxative for several months longer as a form of insurance against a relapse caused by hard stools.

Types of bulk laxative are as follows.

   Colloids. These may be derived from dried fruits, marine algae, mucilages, acacia, tragacanth, or psyllium.[1] However, the version most easily used is methyl cellulose in the form of 'Cologel' (prescribed as methyl cellulose liquid 450). This is a fluid gel which is palatable if kept cool but tends to adopt a rather offensive slimy quality when warmer. This rather disgusting appearance may, paradoxically, increase its acceptability with children who take it from bravado! Those with more discerning palates may prefer tablets ('Celevac'). These agents are best given two to three times daily, with plenty of water.

Lactulose. This is a synthetic disaccharide which is poorly absorbed from the gastrointestinal tract and so reaches the colon where it provides nutrients for the lactobacilli and low molecular weight organic acids; lactic acid and formic acid are formed. The stool, therefore, retains water osmotically and, in addition, the bacterial solid content is increased. A three-week trial of lactulose in mild constipation showed a similar effect to senna,[2] with less colic and diarrhoea in the lactulose group. However, in children with a degree of megarectum lactulose is rarely sufficiently effective without the addition of a period on stimulant laxatives. Lactulose is a useful adjunct to increasing fluids for babies with constipation. In older children it may make the overflow soiling wetter than when methyl cellulose is used. However, it is more easily tolerated by children than methyl cellulose and so is a valuable second-line softener.

Faecal softeners

The bulk laxatives are effective for maintaining the production of soft stool but not as effective in softening hard stools which are already present as those described below.

Mineral oil (liquid paraffin) was a traditional remedy to soften hard, retained stools but the chronic use of this led to interference with the absorption of lipid-soluble vitamins (A, D, and K). The additional risks of inhalation lipid pneumonia, inclusion in the reticulo-endothelial system, and local problems of greasy liquid faecal soiling has discouraged its use.[3]

Docusate (dioctyl sodium sulphosuccinate) is an emulsifying agent and is used as a wetting and dispersing agent. There has been some concern that if used with other medication over a long period it may increase the mucosal uptake of these drugs and, possibly, other toxins. However, it appears safe in practice and fulfils a valuable role when large faecal masses are palpable on abdominal examination. There is also evidence that docusate increases colonic secretion, adding more fluid to the stool as well as breaking up the faecal masses.[4] From a historical viewpoint the bile-like emulsifying activity of docusate is reminiscent of Avicenna's claim that it is the bilious humour which is sensed by the rectum to provide the sensation of the need to defaecate.[5]

Saline cathartics

Magnesia is often recommended to mothers as a gentle purgative in the form of Milk of Magnesia. The effect is by an osmotic action in the intestinal lumen. In too high a dose, and when sodium or potassium salts are used, there is a real risk of absorbing them, resulting in heart failure or hypernatraemia in young infants.

Sodium picosulphate is probably the safest ('Laxoberal') and is less harsh than the sodium picosulphate and magnesium citrate mix in 'Picolax'. Once the stool has been softened with docusate (given as 2 ml/kg body weight/24 hours of Dioctyl Paediatric), a convenient method is to give a dose of Laxoberal (5 ml 2–5 years, 7.5 ml 5–10 years, and 10 ml older than 10 years) on Saturday mornings and a repeat dose six hours later if no stool has been passed. If there is no success then a repeat dose on Sunday could be tried. It is wise to avoid regular medication with sodium picosulphate because of the sodium load, but once a week seems reasonable.

'Golytely' (sodium,potassium sulphate,bicarbonate, poly-ethylene glycol solution) is effective, if given with sufficient water, in clearing the colon without producing electrolyte disturbance.[6] Younger children may not be able to take sufficient volume of fluid and it should be used with caution. Sometimes nasogastric administration is advised but this brings into question whether an enema, given under adequate sedation, would not be less invasive.

Stimulant laxatives

Castor oil contains the triglyceride of ricinoleic acid and works on the small intestine. This is a disadvantage as it may affect the absorption of nutrients and so is not currently in use.

Phenolphthalein is still used in spite of its risk of allergic rashes, and more rarely Stevens–Johnson syndrome and lupus erythematosis. It is found in 'Ex-Lax' chocolate and easily available in chemist shops. Bisacodyl ('Dulcolax') is chemically very similar to phenolphthalein, but safer. It is absorbed, glucuronated in the liver, and then enters the gut again to be active when deglucuronated. The diacetyl form has a direct effect on the gut and so can be used in suppository form. Unfortunately, suppositories are very easily prescribed but very traumatic for the child to receive and particularly stressful for the parents to administer.[7] They, like enemata, should be used when all else fails and preferably with sedation.

The anthraquinone laxatives are cascara, senna, and danthron. They reach the large intestine via the lumen and the circulation. They are hydrolysed in part, by bacterial action and their effect on the large bowel occurs between 6 and 24 hours after ingestion. They are all subject to laxative abuse in adults[8] and may cause toxic degeneration of myenteric plexuses and hence interference with colonic motility.[9] However, senna appears to be the most free of dangerous side effects. No myenteric damage has been observed on prolonged exposure of mice to 'Senokot',[10] although it has been observed when very large doses of senna are given parenterally.[11] This was not confirmed using the purified sennosides A and B found in standardized senna ('Senokot'). Danthron was withdrawn because of possible carcinogenic properties in massive doses in animals when it was tested as a food colouring.

Senna is one of the most widely used stimulant laxatives and is effective in establishing more regular defaecation.[12-14] It is chemically similar to rhubarb (sennosides E and F) and is derived from the leaflets of the *Cassia augustiflora* or *acutiflora* plant. It requires the colonic bacteria to activate the sennosides by metabolizing the sugar groups.

Mistakes are frequently made in using senna for the treatment of chronic constipation.

- Using senna before complete evacuation of old, retained stools leads to abdominal colic and an increase in overflow soiling.

- Used too frequently and ignoring the time lapse from ingestion to action (usually 12-24 hours in children). A daily or alternate day dose is to be preferred to any other regime.

- Using senna for too short a time, giving insufficient opportunity for the bowel habit to become established and the child's confidence to consolidate.

- Not warning children and parents that a year or more on senna may be necessary.

● Not using methyl cellulose or lactulose to maintain a soft but bulky stool.

If these errors are avoided senna can be very helpful in childhood constipation. As Shakespeare put it: 'What rhubarb, senna, or what purgative drug, would scour these English . . .' (*Macbeth* Act V, Scene iii), or Robert Burton in 1621: 'a wonderful herb against melancholy. It scours the blood, lightens the spirits, shakes off sorrow, a most profitable medicine.'

Enemata

A sudden increase in rectal filling will lead to a strong rectal contraction and reflex relaxation of the anal sphincter. An enema will achieve this and evacuate a rectal faecal mass. Phosphate or microenemata are effective in most children but at the cost of discomfort, embarrassment, or fear. Sedation (such as temazepam) or gentle and expert persuasion is essential. Many children have life-long fears induced by being violently held down for an enema.[15] Sometimes, adolescents can be shown how to administer their own enemata. This puts the control back in their hands and can result in acceptance by a number who would have previously rejected the idea. If the enema seems to be necessary it is worth considering whether an evacuation under anaesthetic would not be more humane, more complete, and allow a simultaneous anal dilatation.

References

1. Gray, H. and Tainter, M. L. (1941). Colloid laxatives available for clinical use. *Am. J. Dig. Dis.* 8, 130–9.
2. Perkin, J. M. (1977). Constipation in childhood: a controlled comparison between lactulose and standardised senna. *Curr. med. Res. Opin.* 4, 540–3.
3. Becker, G. L. (1952). The case against mineral oil. *Am. J. Dig. Dis.* 19, 344–8.
4. Clayden, G. S. (1978). Disodium sulphosuccinate in constipation. *Lancet* ii, 787.

5. Cameron-Gruner, O. (1930). *A treatise on the canon of medicine of Avicenna*. Luzac & Co., London.
6. Tolia, V., Fleming, S., and Dubois, R. S. (1984). Use of 'Golytely' in children and adolescents. *J. ped. Gastro. Nutr.* 3, 468–70.
7. Clayden, G. S. (1981). In condemnation of the suppository in childhood. *Lancet* i, 273.
8. Rutter, R. and Maxwell, D. (1976). Diseases of the alimentary system. Constipation and laxative abuses. *Br. med. J.* ii, 997–1000.
9. Cummings, J. H. (1974). Laxative abuse. *Gut* 15, 758–766.
10. Douthwaite, A. H. and Goulding, R. (1957). Action of senna. *Br. med. J.* ii, 1414–15.
11. Smith, B. (1968). Effect of irritant purgatives on the myenteric plexus in man and in the mouse. *Gut* 9, 139–43.
12. Campbell-Mackie, M. (1959). The treatment of bowel dysfunction in infants and young children. *The Practitioner* 183, 732–6.
13. Dubow, E. (1960). Constipation in infants and children. *Arch. Ped. N. Y.* 261–7.
14. Clayden, G. S. and Lawson, J. O. N. (1976). Investigation and management of long standing chronic constipation in childhood. *Arch. Dis. Childh.* 51, 918–23.
15. Pinkerton, P. (1958). Psychogenic megacolon in children: the implications of bowel negativism. *Arch. Dis. Childh.* 33, 371–80.

8. Investigations

RADIOLOGY

Radiology is generally not indicated in uncomplicated cases of constipation. Where constipation is severe and of long standing, or if the diagnosis is uncertain, it may give valuable information about the pathology or anatomy.

Indications for radiological investigations in constipation are as follows:

1. Obstructive constipation, i.e. Hirschsprung's disease etc.

2. Evaluation of a megarectum.

3. Exclusion of other causes, i.e. nephrocalcinosis, renal calculi, etc.

4. Post-operative assessment, i.e. post-Svenson repair, etc.

5. Severe abdominal pain?

Checking for spina bifida occulta with X-rays of the spine in patients who only present with faecal incontinence is not indicated. Spina bifida occulta does not appear to give rise to faecal incontinence as the only symptom, and if it is thought likely that the incontinence is related to spinal dysraphism then urinary symptoms or lower-limb neurological signs would be expected.

Types of X-rays used in assessment of a constipated child are:

- Plain abdominal film.

- Barium studies; enemata, follow-through studies.

- Transit studies.

Plain abdominal films are not very helpful in diagnosis of faecal retention. There are no studies relating severity of constipation/faecal retention with degree of faecal loading, as judged by plain abdominal X-rays. Simple abdominal palpation and/or rectal examination usually gives sufficient information about the severity of retention, thus making radiological investigations superfluous. However, some children are difficult to examine abdominally. They can have a large, soft abdomen with considerable quantities of soft faeces in the abdomen and pelvis, or a hard, tense abdomen with hard faeces distributed throughout the abdominal cavity. In these patients plain abdominal X-rays may be helpful to confirm one's clinical impression.

Barium enemata are often carried out in constipated children with severe functional problems, in order to outline the rectum and confirm whether a megarectum is present. Their value is unclear.[1] The actual size of the rectum can be evaluated in this way[2] and useful information about the post-surgical rectum is obtained. Follow-through studies give information about the large intestine and its size, and are useful in the assessment of Hirschsprung's disease and other neuronal disorders of the hind gut, where extensive bowel dilatation may be seen.

Radiology with radiopaque markers in the evaluation of gastrointestinal (mouth to anus) transit time has been used as an assessment of constipation both in adults and children.[3,4] The patient ingests a number of radiopaque polyethylene pellets (usually 20) 2, 3, or 5 mm in diameter on day one. In adults, serial abdominal plain films, taken at 48–96 hours, will show the distribution of the pellets within the bowel. In children this is probably not ethical but one X-ray at 24–72 hours as well as X-rays of all stools passed during the trial is possible. In children it may be more appropriate to X-ray the stools only, thus avoiding irradiation of the abdomen. With this method it has been found that whole-gut transit is prolonged in constipated children.

Transit-time studies involving radiopaque markers in constipated children have not answered the basic question of whether delayed transit is the effect of faecal stasis, which in chronically constipated children is usually well-established over many years, or whether it is a reflection of an intrinsic intestinal motility disorder.

RECTAL BIOPSY

Histological and histochemical information is obtained through rectal biopsies. This is the only definite way of diagnosing Hirschsprung's disease and other, related neuronal disorders of the hind gut. Suctional biopsy of the mucosa and sub-mucosa gives information about the presence or absence of ganglial cells in the superficial nerve plexuses. False-negative results are rare but possible. Deeper, or full-thickness, biopsies give information about other abnormalities of both the myenteric (Auerbach's plexus) and the submucous (Meissner's) nerve plexuses.

Conventional histology shows the absence of ganglion cells and large nerve trunks between muscle layers and in the sub-mucosal part of the bowel wall. The nerve trunks are strongly positive for acetylcholinesterase and this appearance is characteristic of Hirschsprung's disease.[5] The normal adrenergic nerve arrangement is absent in affected bowel segments in Hirschsprung's disease. Ultra structural examination of Schwann cell bundles shows that the number of axons per bundle is increased but that otherwise they look normal.

In hypoganglionosis a few small ganglia are seen, with acid phosphatase staining on full-thickness biopsy. Acetylcholinesterase staining on superficial biopsy shows paucity of nerves in the submucosa.[4]

In hyperganglionosis, giant ganglia and hyperplasia of the plexuses are seen with moderate elevation of acetylcholinesterase activity in the nerve fibres.

With full-thickness biopsies, detailed histochemical analysis is possible. This involves acid phosphatase, acetylcholinesterase, and catecholamines.

Acid phosphatase—very useful in hypoganglionosis, allows pictorial assessment of ganglion cells in the inter-myenteric zone; full-thickness biopsy.

Acetylcholinesterase—shows ganglion cells and cholinesterase positive nerves; superficial and full-thickness biopsy.

Catecholamine fluorescence—gives information about the distribution of the adrenergic nerves; full-thickness biopsy.

ANORECTAL MANOMETRY

Anorectal manometry is now well-established as a standard investigation of functional disorders of the anorectum. Its main role is in the evaluation of children with severe constipation where the diagnosis of Hirschsprung's disease and other hind gut, neuronal disorders needs to be excluded. Its diagnostic accuracy is similar to that of a rectal biopsy in the diagnosis of Hirschsprung's disease, except during the new-born period when both false negative and positive results may be obtained.[6] If a delay of a few days is allowed the accuracy of this investigation increases to 98 per cent. The anorectal reflex may not be fully developed in the first 48 hours of life, which probably accounts for this. The role of anorectal manometry alone in the assessment of primary referred children with functional constipation and soiling remains uncertain. However, taken in conjunction with other forms of assessment it gives valuable information about the function of the anorectum.

Anorectal manometry can be performed either with air- or water-filled balloons placed in the anorectum, or with open-ended water-perfused catheters which are gradually withdrawn through the anal canal while the pressure is measured. We are accustomed to the former technique. An air-filled rectal balloon of maximal capacity is placed in the rectum. It is on the end of a 14-cm anal probe (see Fig. 5). On the stalk of the probe there are three small water-filled sensor balloons used for

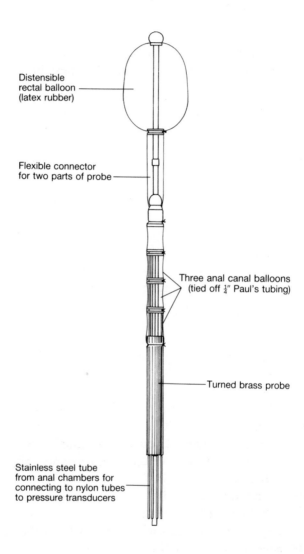

Distensible
rectal balloon
(latex rubber)

Flexible connector
for two parts of probe

Three anal canal balloons
(tied off ¼″ Paul's tubing)

Turned brass probe

Stainless steel tube
from anal chambers for
connecting to nylon tubes
to pressure transducers

Fig. 5a

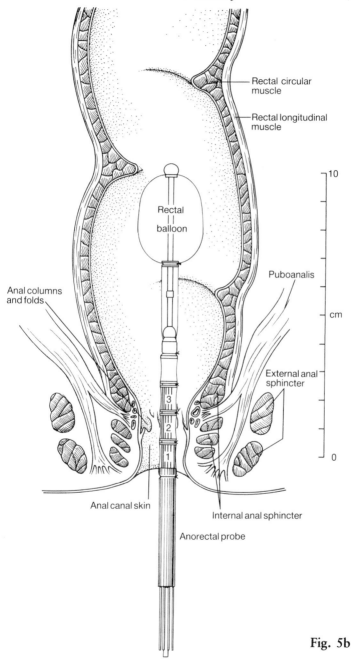

Rectal circular muscle

Rectal longitudinal muscle

Rectal balloon

Anal columns and folds

Puboanalis

External anal sphincter

Anal canal skin

Internal anal sphincter

Anorectal probe

10

cm

0

Fig. 5b

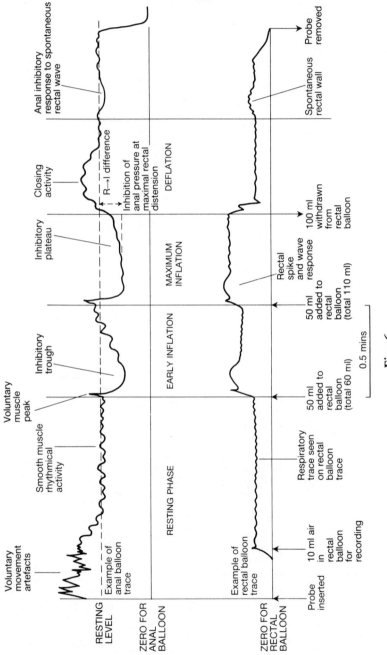

Fig. 6

measuring the pressure in the anal canal, at 1-cm intervals. The outermost anal balloon measures the pressure in the first cm of the anal canal, the second balloon measures pressure in the second cm, and the third balloon in the third cm of the anal canal. The internal sphincter activity is most strongly detected in the second cm and the external sphincter in the first cm. The balloons on the anal probe are connected to pressure transducers, which in turn are connected to a computer, and the anorectal manometry trace is displayed on a monitor screen (see Fig. 6).

Ideally, the procedure is carried out without any sedation, since it is extremely well tolerated. The patient lies on their left side and the probe is inserted. It is important that the probe is held firmly in place and not moved during the procedure. Air is injected into the rectal balloon until the patient can discern the rectal distension. The volume which the patient is first aware of corresponds to the rectal sensation. Gradually, the rectal volume is increased until the maximal tolerable volume is reached. During rectal distension the recto-anal inhibitory reflex is normally displayed on the monitor screen. This is absent in Hirschsprung's disease. The following parameters can be measured with anorectal manometry: mean, maximal, and minimal anal resting pressures; anorectal inhibitory response threshold (volume required to cause a certain fall in anal tone); rectal compliance (rectal distensibility); rectal sensation; ability to defaecate the rectal balloon; ability to squeeze with the external anal sphincter/pelvic floor muscles; anal rhythmical activity assessment (waves/minute, amplitudes). The procedure takes 20–30 minutes and requires minimal preparation. The patient should not be faecally loaded. No anal therapy (enemata, suppositories, manual evacuation of faeces) should have been carried out for at least three days before the procedure and no stimulant laxatives given for 36 hours. If the patient is grossly faecally loaded this should be evacuated well before the investigation.

In children with constipation high,[7,8] normal,[9] or low[10] anal pressures have been reported, the inhibitory reflex threshold appears to be increased,[7] and rectal compliance has been reported as normal[11] or increased.[1] Anal rhythmical activity (generated by the internal anal sphincter) appears to be characterized by slow anal waves in severely constipated children compared to normal children.[12] These are generated low in the anal canal.[13] During defaecation, paradoxical contraction of the external anal sphincter has been found on manometry in those patients that soil badly.[14] In adults, results of anorectal manometry do not seem to vary from one day to another in the same patient.[15] This indicates that the reason for the discrepancies in results reported from studies in children is probably largely due to the different types of equipment used.

References

1. Patriquin, H., Martelli, H., and Devroede, G. (1978). Barium enema in chronic constipation: is it meaningful? *Gastroenterology* 75, 619–22.
2. Meunier, P., Louis, D. and Jaubert de Beaujeu, M. (1984). Physiologic investigations of primary chronic constipation in children: comparison with the barium enema study. *Gastroenterology* 87, 1351–7.
3. Hinton, J. M. and Lennard-Jones, J. E. (1969). A new method for studying gut transit times using radioopaque markers. *Gut* 10, 842–7.
4. Cummings, J. H., Jenkins, D. J. A., and Wiggins, H. S. (1976). Measurement of the mean transit time of dietary residue through the human gut. *Gut* 17, 210–18.
5. Howard, E. R. and Garrett, J. R. (1984). Hirschsprung's disease and other neuronal disorders of the hindgut. In *Neonatal gastroenterology. Contemporary Issues*, (ed. M. S. Tanner and J. G. Stocks). Intercept Ltd, Newcastle upon Tyne.
6. Boston, V. E. and Scott, J. E. S. (1976). Anorectal manometry as a diagnostic method in the neonatal period. *J. ped. Surg.* 11, 9–16.

7. Meunier, P., Marechal, J. M., and Jaubert de Beaujeu, M. (1979). Rectoanal pressures and rectal sensitivity studies in chronic childhood constipation. *Gastroenterology* 77, 330–6.
8. Kaya, I. S., Dilmen, U., and Ceyhan, M. (1988). Rectal and anal pressure profile in constipated children. *Lancet* ii, 1198–9.
9. Suzuki, H., Amano, S., Honzumi, M. *et al.* (1980). Rectoanal pressure and rectal compliance in constipated infants and children. *Z. Kinderchir.* 29, 330–6.
10. Reuter, I. and Kaiser, G. (1976). Betrachtungen zum anorektalen druckprofil. *Helv. Paediatr. Acta* 31, 141–8.
11. Cucchiara, S., Coremans, G., Staiano, A., *et al.* (1984). Gastrointestinal transit time and anorectal manometry in children with fecal soiling. *J. ped. Gastroent. Nutr.* 3, 545–50.
12. Clayden, G. S. (1988). Is constipation in childhood a neurodevelopmental abnormality? In *Disorders of gastrointestinal motility in childhood*, (ed. P. J. Milla). John Wiley and Sons Ltd, Chichester.
13. Hancock, B. D. (1976). Measurement of anal pressure and motility. *Gut* 17, 645–51.
14. Wald, A., Chandra, R., Chiponis, D., and Gabel, S. (1986). Anorectal function and continence mechanisms in childhood encopresis. *J. ped. Gastroent. Nutr.* 5, 346–51.
15. Rogers, J., Laurberg, S., Misiewicz, J. J., Henry, M. M., and Swash, M. (1989). Anorectal physiology validated: a repeatability study of the motor and sensory tests of anorectal function. *Br. J. Surg.* 76, 607–9.

9. Surgical treatments

ANAL DILATATION

Anal dilatation is an old method of treating constipation. In babies and infants it can be carried out by inserting a well-lubricated little finger and holding it in place for a few minutes. This may have to be done on one or two occasions and is often sufficient to relieve mild problems of constipation.[1] It should not be done if anal fissures are present. In older children anal dilatation is carried out under a general anaesthetic. The anus is gently stretched by both index fingers until both middle fingers can be inserted as well. The stretch should not be forced and should last several minutes.

Anal dilatation is usually reserved for those patients where constipation is resistant to standard management.[2] In the opinion of the authors it should be carried out sooner rather than later and not be withheld for many years. It is unclear whether anorectal manometry plays a role in predicting where or when anal dilatation is indicated. One anal dilatation has a success rate of 50 per cent in relieving, or markedly improving, constipation and soiling. If repeated once the success rate improves still further to 80 per cent.[2]

Anal dilatation can be used as follows:

1. Useful in babies and infants. One little finger inserted. One or two dilatations required. No general anaesthetic needed.

2. In older children general anaesthetic required. Up to four fingers inserted. May have to be repeated.

3. Carry out sooner rather than later if no response to therapy.

SPHINCTEROTOMY

This consists of a division of the lower third of the internal sphincter. It is divided up to the level of the dentate line. It is usually reserved for those patients with intractable constipation where anal dilatation has been unsuccessful. As with anal dilatation it is not known whether internal anal sphincter pressure or tone is higher in those requiring this form of treatment.

ANOPLASTY

This operation may be indicated in those patients with severe anterior anal displacements, ectopic anus, covered anus, low types of imperforate anus, etc. Anal cut-back with positioning of the anal orifice more posteriorly on the perineum facilitates normal defaecation.

COLECTOMY

These operations are required for Hirschsprung's disease and related conditions.[3] In the Swenson manoeuvre the whole aganglionic segment is removed with an anastomosis at the anus. This is an extensive operation, not well-tolerated by babies and infants, and therefore a preliminary colostomy above the aganglionic segment is carried out first with later corrective surgery in these patients. In the Duhamel operation the ganglionic proximal colon is brought down, posterior to the aganglionic rectum, which is not resected, and the two are connected by side-to-side anastomosis. This procedure has particular merit for those with aganglionosis of the entire colon. In the Soave procedure the aganglionic rectal musculature is left in place but the rectal mucosa is removed and the normal peristaltic ganglionic segment brought down through the rectal muscular cuff.

In very short-segment Hirschsprung's disease extended anal sphincterotomy is often effective.

If the anal sphincters are poorly developed and/or damaged further during surgery, faecal incontinence may have to be accepted. The role of biofeedback in improving incontinence in these patients is uncertain.

References

1. Harris, L. E., Corbin, P. F., and Hill, J. R. (1953). Anorectal rings in infancy: incidence and significance. *Pediatrics* **13**, 59–63.
2. Clayden, G. S. and Lawson, J. O. N. (1976) Investigation and management of longstanding chronic constipation in childhood. *Arch. Dis. Childh.* **51**, 918–23.
3. Filston, H. C. (1986). *Textbook of surgery. The biological basis of modern surgical practice*, 13th edn. (ed. D. C. Sabiston). W. B. Saunders & Company, Philadelphia.

10. Psychological management

It is helpful to list the main areas which need consideration in the psychological management of the constipated child. Most of the reports from child psychiatrists and psychologists have focused on the child with soiling or encopresis,[1-4] but some have dealt with the stool-withholding behaviour.[5,6]

RECOGNIZING THE PSYCHOLOGICAL ASPECTS

A review of Figure 3 from page 58, concentrating on the psychological aspects shows that the difficulties of the child and family can be seen as follows:

- fear of anal pain;

- confusion by child and family about why the bowel problem is happening;

- embarrassment related to soiling;

- shame of disappointing family;

- confusion about degree of deliberate control of bowels or soiling;

- anger in response to pressure to perform what is feared;

- anger in response to coercion to control what is beyond control;

- despair in the failure of treatment regimes;

- withdrawal or sinking into helplessness;

- dissociation from bowel sensations and activities;

- abdication of responsibilities for bowel activities.

Failure to provide adequate expert help and explanation will lead to sabotage of potentially helpful treatments, deterioration of behaviour as physical symptoms alter, and it can destabilize family relationships which are so often built around the child's problem. The real stressors in the child's life are thus missed, increasing the stress through inappropriate behaviour-modification techniques and missing any 'Munchhausen by proxy' situations. Similarly, a strictly focused and isolated psychological input may take a misguided direction if it is not integrated with physical treatment. Resistance to psychological help may develop if persuasive-training techniques are introduced before the child is physically able to succeed.

SPECTRUM OF PSYCHOLOGICAL HELP

The following is a spectrum of psychological approaches (which should be undertaken by the paediatrician and nurses, who will seek advice and help from psychologists, psychiatrists, and therapists as they find necessary; possibly increasing as we descend the spectrum):

1. Careful explanation of the pathophysiology (demystifying).

2. Assessment of the significance of the condition for child and family.

3. Support to child and family to help with acknowledged chronicity of problem.

4. Support to professionals at frustratingly slow progress and set backs.

5. Use of behaviour-modification methods.

6. Agreeing a contract for toilet training and incentives.

7. Involvement of family in therapy programme.

8. Involvement of in-patient facilities.

9. Individual psychotherapy—play, art, music, eurythmy.

10. Longer in-patient training programmes.

11. Alternative placement outside family.

Demystifying

This can be achieved by carefully explaining the factors leading to the problem and by mapping out the areas of difficulty in a simplified chart, like Fig. 3. This should also clarify the various investigations and actions, and reduce the chance of the child feeling that the tests or treatments are punishments. By sharing this model of management with colleagues, the multidisciplinary approach is facilitated.

Support

The child and family need a great deal of reassurance that the protracted nature of the bowel problems does not indicate a hopeless, endless condition. There is a danger that encouragement can be misunderstood as not taking their problem seriously enough. A tactful prediction of the stages of future improvement, but avoiding a fixed time-scale, may help.

Practical assistance

Practical assistance in coping with the faecal incontinence is essential. Children can be given discrete 'survival packs' to take to school, containing cleaning materials, clean pants, and a plastic bag for soiled clothes. Parents can be given help through specific charities to finance the purchase of a washing machine and possible replacement of damaged clothes. An attendance allowance may be available for certain cases. At home, families should be advised to provide a 'secret bucket' for soiled clothes, so that the child can dispose of what they see as evidence of failure, with the minimum of notice and shame. It is vital that this bucket is discreetly hidden from anyone likely to use its existence as a focus for teasing. Parents must also be prevented from using 'the bucket' as a symbol of the child's failure.

It is essential that the whole multidisciplinary team follows an agreed directional policy in the advice and management offered.

Support to professionals

This is also an important feature. The chronic and unglamorous nature of constipation and incontinence, the level of despair in the children and families, and the apparent lack of real progress, all combine to undermine the morale of staff. Team meetings and regular feedback can help. The nursing staff in children's wards or in the community are usually at the front line, treating the child during the worst of the problems and rarely seeing the child who has been discharged from the follow up clinic 'cured'. Feedback reports of ultimate successes are therefore essential. It is usually the consultant who receives the 'thank you' letters and long term progress reports. Reviewing these letters in the multidisciplinary team and inviting members from the wards and community to the follow-up clinics will inevitably improve morale. There is a strong argument for concentrating children with bowel problems within a single clinic. Individual children and their families may benefit from the effect that the progress of the preceding child has had on the doctor, by creating a generally positive and encouraging approach.

Contracts and incentives

These are important tools but must be detailed. At times, when the family's anxiety is producing excessive hostility to the physical problems, a calm discussion, reiterating the need for a structured approach to the practical steps useful in overcoming some of the difficulties, can temper the emotional heat with intellectual coolness. It is very useful to draw up a list of the more annoying features.

For example: hiding soiled clothes, avoiding using the lavatory, refusing medication, mocking, anger, or shaming by the family when the child soils, family jokes about the 'stinky' child are out of place. Contracts can be drawn up with the family to prevent such responses. Help from the psychologist may be useful here but all those involved must understand the contracts and help the reinforcement of any incentive scheme. A simple star chart, worked out and agreed by the child, family, and psychologist can be extremely effective. If stars alone are insufficient reward they can be used as tokens towards a more tangible gift. The main danger in using these methods is in designing a system in which the child is bound to fail. It is vital to ensure medically that the child is physically able to achieve given targets before starting incentive charts.

Family 'therapy'

It is impossible to use any of the above methods without the full involvement of the family. Family meetings are essential in implementing contracts and incentives and explaining the interaction of the physiological, pharmacological, and psychological aspects. However, it may become clear that the dynamics operating in the family are highly complex and deeply woven into the bowel problem. For example, there may be concealed psychiatric illness in the family which is using the child's symptoms to maintain some stability. The threat of change in the family by the child losing the bowel problem may lead to conscious or unconscious sabotage of the treatments offered. The involvement of the parents in trying to cope with the child's problem, however stressful, may be the only element in their lives which they have in common, and they may be naturally anxious to maintain it. Sometimes the child is made a scapegoat or favoured as a result of the problem. Sometimes the bowel problem is a defensive reaction to an abusive situation in the family. More rarely, the problem is created or maintained by a parent with the Munchhausen syndrome (see page 90).

All these and many other possibilities must be considered, and may appear, during family sessions. The team is clearly dealing with a potentially explosive situation, however, and so great care and skill is required by the professionals, and family therapy should never be entered into casually. Most professionals insist on conducting family sessions in pairs, or working with other professionals viewing the proceedings through one-way mirrors, closed circuit television, or video, as advisors.

Individual therapy

Sometimes the child with severe constipation and soiling becomes so dissociated from the offending parts of their body or so low in self esteem that individual therapy is essential. In all children there is an attempt to engage by the professionals, to explain and reassure, but in the very withdrawn or, more commonly, very dissociated child other methods may be necessary. It is a common experience that stress has a direct effect on the bowels and this has been confirmed experimentally.[7] Individual psychotherapy using play or drawing may help the child to establish a link in communication. We have found two methods, art therapy and eurythmy, particularly helpful in children who appear to be managing reasonably well on the surface but in whom the deeper emotional turmoil is denied, despite its having a physiological effect.

The aim of art therapy is to give the child an opportunity, in a safe one-to-one situation, to express these deeper and physiologically disturbing emotions in a more creative way. Trained art therapists appear to do for the emotionally crippled child what the physiotherapist does for those with physical disability. By providing a safe and reassuring space for the child, they can be helped to experience the movement of these emotions through the creative medium, without conscious or intellectual screening of their content. This free flow of feelings can panic the child unless carefully managed by the therapist, but can be a powerful means of discharging some of the blocked emotions.[8]

Eurythmy also appears to help children in whom there appears to be a disruption of the integration of the emotions, physiology, and conscious perception of the bowel activity. Eurythmy, an art of movement, is based on the work of Steiner and involves a regulated relationship of the individual with their will in movement and gesture. Highly trained therapists take the child, individually or in small groups, through movement linked with the spoken word in a series of sessions tailored to the child's need in terms of self esteem, self awareness, and expressiveness.[8]

It is obviously very difficult to evaluate such individually designed therapies but it is clear from experience that a number of children who were previously worn down and despairing by their distressing symptoms have been able to lift themselves sufficiently for the other methods described to help.

In-patient treatment

This is sometimes necessary to consolidate the out-patient treatment regimes. No success can be achieved by a short burst of training in hospital unless there is a fundamental change in the child and family's attitude to the problem, which will continue after discharge. Follow-up sessions are essential. During the hospital admission it should be possible for the children to meet others who have been experiencing the stress of bowel problems. Children's groups and separate parent groups can be valuable but potentially explosive. These should be run by trained staff who are supported by the larger multidisciplinary team. If parent groups are not properly planned and constituted, spontaneous liaisons develop and there can be 'contamination' between the parents, where assumptions that their children have identical diseases because their symptoms are similar can lead to misunderstanding. This may lead to parents demanding an escalation of the physical treatments which appeared to have revolutionized the problems in another family.

It appears to be far more acceptable to parents to discover their child has Hirschsprung's disease than a more minor form of megarectum which has led to a similar reduction of health for mainly psychological reasons. This is not surprising as it is easier to visualize the organic defects and to discuss the intricacies of operations with family and friends than to explore the regions of shame, guilt, family dynamics, and the physical effects of emotional stress. This parental denial of the psychological elements may force the paediatrician and nurses into far more of a psychotherapeutic role than they feel qualified to provide. Here the multidisciplinary team should support them until the denial recedes, as it usually does unless too much pressure is imposed on the family in the early stages. Then, the denial is reinforced with a keen sense of threat to their autonomy and leads to consolidation of the rejection of the psychological aspects of the model. However, the paediatricians and nurses should be vigilant for the parents who, in their desperation for help through physical means, sabotage simple treatments and even falsify reports of symptoms. This group may be called 'Munchhausen in desperation syndrome' but will inevitably overlap with the classical 'Munchhausen by proxy' parents who invent factitious symptoms and signs to fool professionals, even into performing major surgery. There is usually a history of multiple operations in the mother and sometimes past psychiatric involvement.

Separation from family

This is the most extreme of the psychological interventions and is restricted to those children who improve steadily in hospital and deteriorate at home. It is usually because the adverse dynamics within the family are too established to alter or the situation is related to child abuse in any of its forms. The emotional abuse of shaming and psychological punishments is often overlooked but is a major element in the deterioration of the child on returning home, or who produces symptoms of extreme distress at home (e.g. obvious delinquent behaviour or running away from home). Physical abuse, often related to soiling is not unusual. This clearly produces a vicious cycle of soiling–punishment–fear–soiling. Sexual abuse is also a cause of severe emotional distress which can present as soiling.[9] Soiling may be a method of trying to repel the abuser or as a result of direct anal trauma. Constipation may be the result of anal pain from buggery or as a method of escaping from the family to hospital. These factors must be weighed against the difficulty of diagnosis in the constipated child where the anal signs can be very misleading.[10,11]

Whatever the original need, the child who is placed away from home may see this as a punishment for the soiling or constipation unless careful explanation and support is given. A misunderstanding like this is likely to lead to a lifelong sense of injustice at being punished for a symptom over which there is no chance of control.

References

1. Richmond, J., Eddy, E., and Garrard, S. (1954). The syndrome of fecal soiling and megacolon. *Am. J. Orthopsychiat.* 24, 391–401.
2. Anthony, E. J. (1957). An experimental approach to the psychopathology of childhood: encopresis. *Br. J. med. Psychol.* 30, 146–75.
3. Pinkerton, P. (1958). Psychogenic megacolon in children: the implications of bowel negativism. *Arch. Dis. Childh.* 33, 371–80.
4. Hersov, L. (1977). Faecal soiling. In *Child psychiatry*, modern approaches, (ed. M. Rutter and L. Hersov). Blackwell Scientific Publications, Oxford.
5. Berg, I. and Vernon-Jones, K. (1964). Functional faecal incontinence. *Arch. Dis. Childh.* 39, 465–72.
6. Buchanan, A. (1990). *Soiling children*. PhD thesis. University of Southampton.
7. Chaudhary, N. A. & Truelove, S. C. (1961). Human colonic motility: Part III: Emotions. *Gastroenterology* 40, 27–36.
8. Frommer, E. A. (1972). *Diagnosis and treatment in clinical child psychiatry*, pp. 179–215. William Heinemann Medical Books, London.

9. Hobbs, C. J. and Wynn, J. M. (1989). Sexual abuse of English boys and girls: the importance of anal examination. *Child Abuse and Neglect* 13, 195–210.
10. Clayden, G. S. (1988). Reflex anal dilatation associated with severe chronic constipation in children. *Arch. Dis. Childh.* 63, 832–6.
11. Butler-Schloss, E. (1987). *Report of the inquiry into child abuse in Cleveland*. Her Majesty's Stationery Office, London.

Appendix. Information booklet for children and parents

The following pages contain the booklet which we hand out routinely to the children attending our special clinics. This has been rigorously edited and criticized by a large number of these children. The language is aimed at a 10–12 year old but it can be read to younger children. This attempt to demystify the subject has succeeded in many cases and has lead other children to frame their questions around particular points in the text. When the booklets are given out a reminder of the individual nature of the problems in that particular child is given.

Readers are invited to photocopy this section of this book for their patients' use, if they feel this may be helpful. This will not infringe the Copyright Laws, unless a charge is made for a copy or an attempt is made to publish the booklet without permission of the authors and Oxford University Press.

SOME INFORMATION ABOUT CHRONIC CONSTIPATION IN CHILDREN

Introduction

We are often asked to explain what is happening inside a child with chronic constipation. This is not easy to answer for two reasons:

(1) No one knows exactly how we learn to control our bowels, nor how that end of the body works.

(2) Every child has an individual form of constipation. Each one has a particular mixture of all the factors which make up the problem.

In this booklet, we try to explain many of the possible factors, and your own individual problem will be caused by some, but not all of these. We hope to find out which are the main ones as you come to the clinic appointments. We will then give you our theory of why the problem is there and suggest the best way of solving it.

Contents

SOME PRACTICAL HINTS

(1) We know that repeated hospital visits are difficult, what with travelling and waiting, so we try to reduce these to a minimum. We know that most children will need to come for at least one year and so we try to spread these appointments out. At first they will be approximately monthly but very soon about three monthly. It is important to be able to keep in touch between these appointments, so we can make small alterations, etc. We try to run a telephone service where we can return your call, or arrange an earlier appointment. Clinics try to be flexible about dates and times, so please alter an appointment, especially if it clashes with something good happening at school. (We sometimes have to alter clinic dates as well.) Some play facilities are available in the clinics, but it is well worth bringing your own toys and books (especially for the grown ups!).

(2) You will probably be given diary sheets to record the medicines given and your progress. Please bring these to clinics and ask for new ones when you are there.

(3) Try to discuss with your local family doctor what is going on if you get the chance. We will write to him at times. He may be asked to prescribe your medicines, as most hospitals cannot give out enough to last the length of time between Out-Patient Clinic visits. It is best to take the empty bottles along to the surgery so the doctors can read the labels, in case they have not received letters from us.

(4) We are happy to write to school doctors or anyone else helping your family, with your permission.

(5) When clinics are arranging special tests or even an In-Patient stay, these arrangements may be complicated. Try and telephone to confirm these dates, if you haven't had official confirmation the week before.

A3

The words we use

It is often embarrassing talking about bowel problems. One added difficulty is the large number of words used for the subject. Here are some of them and their medical terms:

Defaecation—opening the bowels, having a pooh, passing motions, big jobs, doing No. 2, big toilet, going to the loo/lavatory/toilet.

Faeces—stools, poohs, No. 2s, big jobs, plops, bowel motions, (plus those Anglo-Saxon words which may offend some of our readers!).

Most families have their own word for it and it is important we all know what it is when discussing problems.

HOW THE BOWEL WORKS

What are stools?

When we eat, our teeth crush up food until it is soft and we swallow it. When we swallow food, it starts on its journey down a tube (about 26 ft long) from your mouth to your anus (bottom). This long tube (your bowels or gut) gets wider in places, e.g. the stomach. As the food passes along, all the useful parts are absorbed into the blood in the tiny blood vessels running beside the bowel. The blood then carries these 'goodies' to other parts of the body where they are stored, or used to give you energy to run about, to build strong bones, or to make you grow. Gradually all the useful parts are absorbed, leaving just the waste. The last part of the bowel (called the large intestine or large bowel, or colon) allows this waste to move slowly through, and the water is absorbed. You can imagine how important this is in hot countries, especially in deserts. Thus the stool becomes less watery and more formed.

Stools will be different if we eat different things. Some foods leave lots of waste by the time they reach the large bowel—these are called 'high fibre' foods, e.g. apples, peas, potatoes, lettuce, cereals. Some foods contain very little fibre—such as cheese, milk, sweets. If there is too little fibre reaching the large bowel, then stools (poohs) can become rather hard. Fibre helps stools to remain large and soft. If we don't drink enough water or other drinks, the large bowel will do its best to absorb as much water as possible from the stool—it thinks it's in a desert! Thus the stool gets very hard and dry, becoming difficult to pass.

A4

How do we pass stools?

Stools reach the far end of the large bowel (called the rectum). When the stool enters, the rectum seems to feel it arrive there. A message is sent up the nerves to warn you a stool has arrived and you will need to find the loo soon. Another message is sent down to the muscles keeping the anus closed. This message makes the muscles relax slightly and the stool can move further down. When the stool touches the special skin inside the anus, our feeling of wanting to go gets more urgent. These muscles are not directly under our control: they are part of the automatic system which moves food along this tube, from your throat to your anus. Luckily we have some muscles at our bottoms which we can control ourselves, so when the urgent need to pass a stool comes, we can just about hold on for the time it takes to find a loo.

Everybody is different when it comes to the feeling they get from their bottoms, and how easily they can hold on until they find a loo. This difference is the clue as to why some people get constipated (that is, having difficulties in passing stools) and some do not.

Before going into details about this we must know how we learn about the feelings in our bottoms, and what to do about them:

How do children learn to control their bowels?

When babies are fed, as their little stomachs get full, a message is automatically sent down to the rectum. It is as if the stomach were warning the large bowel to empty so as to make room at the top end for milk. For this reason, babies often have stools after feeding. When babies get a feeling from the rectum that it is full, the stool is ready to come out, they automatically relax their bottom muscles, grunt, and push out the stool.

As they grow older, their parents learn to notice when the child (from around the age of two years) is getting this feeling. Quite often the toddler stands quietly as if concentrating and may even go a little red around the eyes, or pale around the nose and lips when s/he is about to go. If the parents manage to put the child on the pot, then the stool will go in the pot and the toddler will see it and notice how pleased Mum and Dad are. He or she will gradually learn that those early feelings coming from the bottom are a sign to sit on the pot which parents get pleased about. It takes months for most children to learn this and sometimes there are problems.

A5

WHY DOES CONSTIPATION HAPPEN?

As we said at the beginning of this booklet, no one child has exactly the same problem as another. There are sorts of constipation which happen more at one age than another. Babies and toddlers may find that their stools are hard to pass. This is often because the child is not having enough water to drink in the day. The stools get dried up and hard. Each day stools are smaller than usual and so it may take two or three days longer for the rectum to fill enough to set off the grunting and straining. Some minor illnesses like a cold or the 'flu will increase the body's need for water and so the stools become harder and less frequent. In some children, when they pass these hard, delayed stools, it hurts. If they are old enough to remember this, the next time they are about to go, they get frightened it will hurt again and so hold on as hard as they can, with their muscles. Unfortunately for them, they have to go some time. By the time they do go—maybe after several days—the stool is very hard and large. This produces pain and once again they learn that defaecating is a bad idea. At a young age they don't understand that they can't just put off going.

A routine develops of being OK for a couple of days, then a day or more of getting feelings of wanting to go. This makes them afraid they will go and so they stand around (or hide) and strain all their bottom muscles to stop going. They often get angry or irritable because they are not feeling too good, what with the feelings coming from their bottoms and the fear that a hard stool will come out and hurt them. Eventually it does come and, if it is hard, it will hurt again, so they are proved right. Naturally the parents are worried that the child must have a motion. They know that all the days of delay are making the stool even harder and larger. They try to help by putting the child on the loo or pot. The last thing the child wants to do is to have a motion and so jumps straight off. As you know, this is bound to lead to a battle; both sides are right, but they have a different understanding of what is going on. Put into words they might say:

CHILD: "Stop it—you are trying to make me have a pooh which will hurt my bottom. You are trying to hurt me!"

PARENT: "Sit there—don't hold on to your pooh or else it will be painful for you another day. Go now—it will be worse later."

A6

Like many battles, a lot of other fights happen as well—'Do as you are told', 'Go away', 'We know best', 'I want to choose for myself'. The battles get hotter when the parents get worried that constipation is making the child ill and they therefore fight harder to save him or her. Fortunately, it is very rare that constipation is dangerous in a child over two years old, but the going off food and looking ill is a worry.

Why does this only happen to some children of this age?

There are several reasons again, and usually the reason for a particular family is a mixture of factors. The size of the rectum varies from child to child—just like there is a difference in how tall you are, or how long your nose is, or what size shoes you take. Some children are born with, or develop, a large rectum. This allows the stools to be stored for a longer time. It may be that a baby with a slightly large rectum will develop a larger one as s/he grows up with constipation. It is probably true that the longer you can hang on to the stools, the larger the rectum is.

Another reason is that some children and parents are more sensitive to worries about stools. Some are more likely to have battles over things like eating, getting dressed, going to bed, etc. If these children are unlucky enough to have a hard stool at some stage, then a battle may develop over this. There is nearly always a bit of this and a bit of that in how constipation develops.

What happens when constipation goes on for a long time?

(We will come to treatment and ways of helping, soon.)

Some children seem to have constipation which goes on and on. Often this is complicated by soiling loose stools into the clothing. This becomes an urgent reason for getting the bowels sorted out, as the soiling can cause great embarrassment. When constipation has been going on for a long time, the rectum is usually large and filled up with hard or soft stools. We can feel how much has built up by abdominal examination (feeling the tummy).

A7

Diagram of the last part of the large bowel

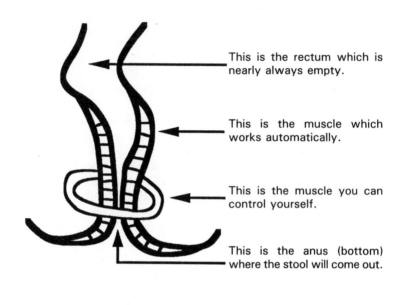

This is the rectum which is nearly always empty.

This is the muscle which works automatically.

This is the muscle you can control yourself.

This is the anus (bottom) where the stool will come out.

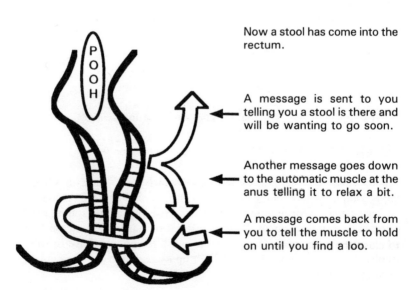

Now a stool has come into the rectum.

A message is sent to you telling you a stool is there and will be wanting to go soon.

Another message goes down to the automatic muscle at the anus telling it to relax a bit.

A message comes back from you to tell the muscle to hold on until you find a loo.

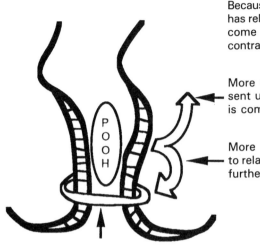

Because the automatic muscle has relaxed a bit, the stool has come lower and the rectum contracts to push it lower still.

More warning messages are sent up to say that the stool is coming out soon.

More messages come down to relax the automatic muscle further.

Your messages to hold on tight with this muscle stop when you find the loo and sit down and relax. (This muscle can only hold on for a short time when the message from the rectum completely relaxes the automatic muscle.)

The rectum contracts and helps push out the stool. You get a feeling that you should push down into your bottom by holding your breath or grunting.

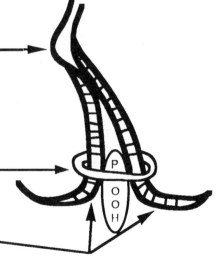

Both the automatic muscle and your controlling muscle are relaxed and the stool comes out easily

These muscles contract afterwards to close the anus again.

Diagram of the last part of the large bowel in chronic constipation

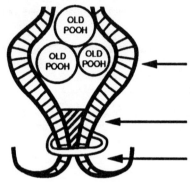

This is the enlarged rectum, pretty full of old stools.

Because it is used to holding heavy stools, the walls are thickened.

There is a little loose stool which passes around the harder stools.

The automatic muscle at the anus is also thickened.

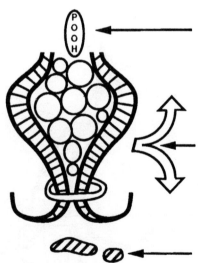

When a new stool comes into the rectum, it is so loaded it doesn't seem to notice its arrival and so no messages are sent up to warn you that another stool has come in.

The rectum churns the old stools about and sometimes sends messages up: but it says that the rectum is quite loaded, but it is not urgent. Sometimes a message is sent down to the automatic muscle, which relaxes only enough to let out some of the soft fluid stools. These seep out, without any feeling and stain the pants.

Because no clear messages are coming up from the rectum, this muscle which we can control ourselves does not squeeze and stop the fluid soiling.

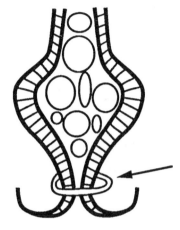

After about 1 to 3 weeks, the rectum gets very loaded, then it starts to give messages which often feel like pain in the tummy. Eventually the automatic muscle gets enough message to relax and let out the giant stool.

The muscle you can control is eventually unable to stop the large stool coming out and it gets so urgent a rush to the loo is needed.

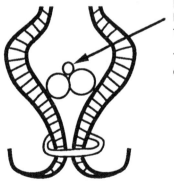

Even after all this, there is still some left, which will be the old stool at the centre of the next giant stool.

Thank goodness that's out but, oh dear, not another blocked loo!

The vicious circles

The first vicious circle is that the distended and enlarged rectum allows a large collection of stools, which makes the rectum grow larger, and so on:

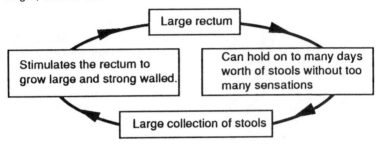

The next vicious circle is that the children who have a dislike of stools (they even dislike the smell of stools, more than children who have not had these problems), so they try as hard as they can not to make stools. This means the stools build up inside and only the fluid, loose stool leaks out. This causes soiling which causes more embarrassment and the child hates stools even more.

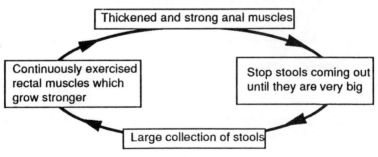

Another vicious cycle is that the muscle wall of the rectum becomes thickened when it is persistently loaded (as if it were an athlete doing weight training). The thickening and strengthening of the muscles also involves the automatic muscles of the anus. This means it takes more messages from the rectum to make it relax and, even then, its thickness does not allow the ordinary sized stools to come down easily.

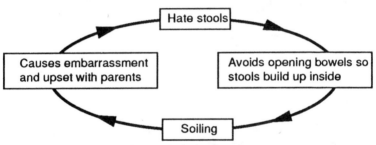

A12

Another circle we discussed earlier is the child who is afraid that a large stool will hurt, and so avoids passing it until it becomes large enough to cause pain:

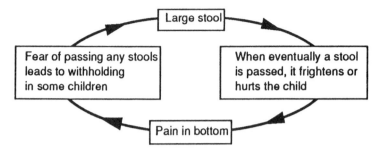

If this becomes a battle area between parent and child, this cycle gets worse.

Another cycle which occurs in chronic constipation, and which will be looked at in the next section, is our diet (what we eat).

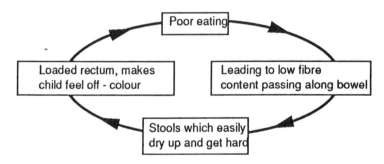

There are many other circles like these, which happen in some children and not in others. These are often connected with the emotional effects of this difficult problem. Again, we must emphasize that every child is different, and not all these cycles happen in every child.

This all sounds very difficult, but keep reading, because we will now show you how many ways we have to help.

A13

1. Food

Some foods have the wrong effect because they tend to slow down the movement of the bowels or fill the child up, so they don't want to eat very much. Milk and sweets (especially sweet milky tea or coffee) do this.

Any food which leaves fibre when it passes through the bowel will help keep stools soft. If the large rectum needs to work on large stools, then high fibre foods will help. The stools will fill up the large rectum within a few days staying soft and so be less likely to hurt.

Food such as these contain lots of fibre:

Cereals like oatmeal porridge, All Bran, Shredded Wheat, Shreddies and Weetabix. Apples and pears with skins, soft fruit, grapes, etc., baked jacket potatoes (skins should be eaten), wholemeal bread, digestive biscuits.

Adequate fluid intake—6–8 cups of liquid a day (everything counts—tea, juice, etc.),

Fruit and vegetables (cooked or uncooked)—root vegetables have higher roughage. The only problem with making changes in the diet is that many of the fibre foods are not very popular with children. This may lead to more disagreements—over meals.

Luckily we have some medicines which provide this sort of roughage, and help keep the stool soft, such as:

Methyl cellulose—Cologel, Celevac, Cellucon.

Bran tablets—Fybranta, Isphagula, Regulan, Metamucil.

Other roughage medicines—Fybogel, Isogel, Inolaxine, Normocol.

Medicines which contain special sugars called 'long sugars' do not get absorbed from the bowel, but stay in the waste from food. When these sugars reach the large bowel, they get eaten by the good germs which we all have there. It may seem unpleasant to you that inside us there are a lot of germs, but these are very useful and some make vitamins to keep us healthy. The others help to keep our stools soft and probably help to keep harmful germs away. Lactulose is the name of one of these sugars and you find this in medicines such as Duphalac and Gatinar.

A14

2. Routines

The body seems to like keeping to regular rhythms—e.g. times of meals, going to bed, waking up, and having a motion. When we have trouble with passing stools apart from keeping the stools soft by having plenty of roughage, we can help by trying regularly. The most likely time to be successful is after eating (just like the babies mentioned on page A5). If you try after every meal, you may find that you occasionally succeed at a particular time in the day. It is worth staying on the loo for ten minutes or more—even if you don't feel like going—especially at those times, and it is worth having a stock of comics there. Sometimes you might pass a small stool and jump off but, if you wait, quite often another comes (try timing when the second one comes!).

3. Medicines

When constipation has been going on a long time, we must find some medicine to help send the stools along faster and make the rectum contract more. Many people use Senokot, mainly because the amount you need can be changed quite safely, and most children like the taste of the syrup. It can also be given as granules or tablets. We advise you to take it only once per day and it is best taken in the evening. It takes quite a long time to work—about 12 to 24 hours. This is because it doesn't work until the good old germs in the large bowel have had a chance to eat some of it. When it starts to work, the muscles in the large bowel start to work more. The stool gets moved about and you sometimes feel this as a feeling that you sometimes want to pass a stool, but often as a funny feeling or even as a slight ache. If you feel any of these, try to pass a stool. When you have had a motion, the Senokot seems to make sure the rectum is really empty and this should help stop what happens in the diagram on page A11.

A15

Senna is a plant which has been used for years to help overcome constipation; here is an old fashioned drawing of the plant from 1646:

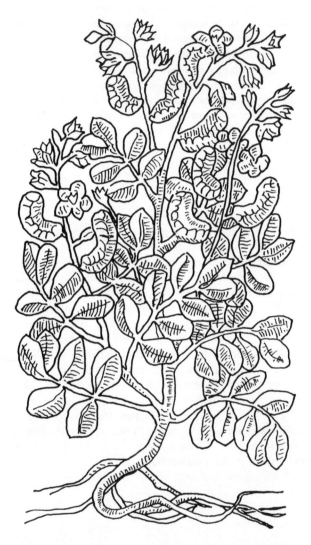

Nowadays the pods from the plant are purified and the Senokot you have is much easier to take. Everyone is individual, and some people do not like Senokot, so we have other medicines which work in a similar way: Normax, Dulcolax.

A16

If you look back at the diagram of the loaded rectum on page A10, you can see that sometimes the large stools clog up at the end of the bowel. Before we can start to use medicines like Senokot, we have to use something to get rid of the hard old stools. If we don't, then powerful medicines like Senokot will just cause discomfort. We try to soften up these stools and 'dissolve' them with Docusate. This medicine has the same effect on stools as washing up liquid has on greasy plates: it helps to loosen the hard stools so they can be passed. Sometimes the stools are so hard they take too long to dissolve and then an enema may be given. This means a small amount of medicine is squirted into the rectum through a small tube passed through the anus. This loosens everything up, makes the rectum very active and helps the stool come out. Usually we don't have to use enemas, but many children have had one by the time they come to a clinic, which is why we tell you about them. Sometimes picosulphate is used to clear out the old stools instead. This is taken by mouth and works in about 6 hours.

It is important that all your medicines are taken regularly. This helps get the body into a rhythm. We often start patients with a week or two of Docusate and then go on to regular Cologel (to keep the stool soft) and use Senokot at night (to keep the bowel moving regularly, and help the rectum shrink down a bit). As you get better, the dose of Senokot can be reduced, perhaps to every other day, and you will gradually need less and less. If you were having 20 mls (four teaspoonfuls) every night, then it is best not to stop this suddenly, but over a couple of weeks, reduce to 15 mls (three teaspoonfuls) or 10 mls (two teaspoonfuls). To help you (and us), the diary sheets give you a space to tick how much you have had. If you take Senokot tablets, one tablet is the same as 5 mls of syrup.

Some children find Cologel difficult to take because, if it warms up it goes thick (a bit like glue!). If you keep it in the fridge, it will stay runny. Another medicine we use is Lactulose, which toddlers and young children take 5 mls of twice a day, and older children take 10 mls twice a day. It is best to keep these going on longer than the Senokot, probably for three to six months, even when you are getting better. This is to stop the constipation happening again, while the rectum is gradually shrinking down to a better size.

4. Special tests

Sometimes we need to do tests to find out exactly what is causing your bowel problem. Usually we get an X-ray picture of your abdomen (tummy) to see where the stools are: we will show you this X-ray. If your bottom problem is quite complicated, and is not getting better, we may carry out other tests.

One test is to put a little balloon in your bottom—you just feel something cold and then you lie there while the machine records things and prints it out on paper. We will show you this tracing and try to explain how your bottom works. This takes about 20 minutes and all you usually notice is the cold feeling as the balloon goes in, or occasionally a feeling that you would like a motion, or nothing at all. What we see looking at the recording, is how well the automatic muscle relaxes. Most children who are old enough to read this (e.g. over seven years old) find the test a bit odd, but certainly not distressing. It is difficult to explain this test to younger children, who are often very frightened of things to do with bottoms and stools, so we do this test under an anaesthetic.

Another test which is sometimes done is a special X-ray called a barium enema. Here a small amount of special liquid is squirted into the anus and X-rays are taken: this shows the shape of the lower bowel. You may have had this test done in the past.

There is one condition we are very careful to look for in all constipated children and this has the name of Hirschsprung's disease. Hirschsprung was a doctor in Denmark during the last century: he described two children who had very severe loading of their rectums. It was later found that the automatic muscles do not relax properly in Hirschsprung's disease. This is because the messages from the bowel above cannot pass to the bowel below because the nerves in the bowel wall are not properly formed. This problem mainly affects babies but, just rarely, we see children who have had trouble with this since they were babies. These children do not get better by taking medicines alone. Our balloon test shows that the automatic muscle of the anus does not relax in children with Hirschsprung's disease. To be sure not to miss any constipated children with this disease, we sometimes do a rectal biopsy. This is usually done under an anaesthetic—a tiny piece of the rectum wall is snipped off and looked at under the microscope. We then count the number of nerves there. If there are too few, an operation is needed to put the constipation right.

A18

As we said earlier, the problem of constipation is not just the shape of the rectum or the anus. Sometimes small physical problems are made worse by worries. So other tests are available to help find out if you have any difficulties at school: a psychologist may see you, or if you are having problems with your speech, a speech therapist.

5. Special help

Sometimes, problems with the bowels upset children and their parents so much that this upset makes the problem last longer. This is another circle which we need to break. We try and help by providing social workers, child psychiatrists, and art therapists. They help in many cases by relieving some fears and misunderstandings. Sometimes children keep their feelings inside them and they need to let them out in order for them to be dealt with. Sometimes the battles going on between the parents and child need someone from the outside to bring about a peace treaty! Often children feel that they will never get better and they need encouraging and praising. Some of them are still not sure that having a motion is a good idea, and they need help to try and be reassured that it is. A stay in the children's ward may help, because they see other children with similar worries. Most families feel they are the only ones with this bowel problem. This is probably true of their neighbourhood, but hospitals see children from quite a large area of England and sometimes from abroad, so there is nearly always someone else in the ward with this problem.

6. When do we need to bring children into hospital?

We have mentioned that sometimes we have to do tests which require anaesthetic, so children have to come into hospital for this. Sometimes we want to see just what the pattern of passing stools is. Occasionally, we cannot clear the stools from the loaded rectum and we need to clear them out under an anaesthetic. We also have learned, from treating children with Hirschsprung's disease, that stretching the troublesome automatic muscle of the anus, under anaesthetic, helps in some cases. We find that giving children with chronic constipation an anal dilatation, as it is called, weakens the automatic anal muscle. You remember that it is the muscle which cannot relax properly and will only let the stool out when the rectum is really loaded. By stretching it under anaesthetic we weaken it and from then on the rectum can empty when it is less loaded. So children find they can go more easily and without pain. One extra value of doing this, is that under anaesthetic we can do the balloon test or a rectal biopsy. We can also check how large the anus is, whether it is in the correct position and at the same time, remove any stools loading the rectum.

This can be done just as a Day Case (staying in for one day only), but we often find a few days stay, preferably with Mum, is better. When children are on the ward, we can see that the medicines are the right ones for them, and that they are happier going to the loo. We may give them a chart on which they can put a star every time they pass a stool in the loo. Often they have had these charts before, but have been unable to go and are disappointed. Now they will be able to go, and will get some stars. After they go home they are advised not to stop their medicines too soon, in case loading should come back and undo some of the good that has been done.

Another bonus for the parents on the children's ward is that they meet other parents whose children have similar problems. Again, please remember that all children are different.

Sometimes children need more than one anal dilatation, or even a small cut into the troublesome muscle (this is called a sphincterotomy). Fortunately, this does not lead to any difficulties with holding the stools normally. The soiling is usually the first problem to disappear with any of these treatments. All the different tests and treatments take time to be performed. Some of the arrangements for these are complicated and may even have to be changed at short notice. We try hard to fit our plans in with yours, so as not to interfere with your holidays or arrange for a test to be done in hospital on your birthday. Please let us know in plenty of time if the dates are not right for you so we can give you another. If you forget to come to an out-patient visit, please telephone and make another appointment—we don't want you to get lost. Sometimes we have to change your appointment, or even delay your coming into hospital, because the wards are full of unexpected emergencies. We realize this is disappointing and are sorry if it happens.

It always seems a long time for children to get over their problems with their bowels. Please don't expect a treatment to work quickly or to be able to come off a medicine after just a few weeks. Most children need to come to their out-patient clinics for at least one year.

When you eventually come off medicines, you won't need to attend routinely but we are still happy to hear from you and happy to give further advice in the future. You may be sent letters or forms to fill in many years after you stop coming, which will ask how you are. These help us find out more about these bowel problems. So if you change your address when you have stopped coming to the clinic, please let us know of your new address. (If you can remember your hospital number, this will also be of help).

A20

If you have managed to read through all this, you will probably have quite a few questions! Please ask them next time you come to your out-patient appointment. It sometimes helps if your parents write any questions down, so you don't forget to ask them when you see us.

G. S. Clayden
V. Agnarsson
London

Index

recto-anal reflex (anorectal reflex)
73, 75, 76
rectosigmoid sphincter 40
reflex
anal dilation 12
anocutaneous 49
anorectal 11
gastrocolic 11
in spinal lesions 51
inhibition 11
refusal, pot or lavatory 34
regurgitation 46
reinforcement 87
rejection 90
relapse 63
relationships, family 31
relief and megarectum 38
renal
calculi 70
tubular acidosis 42
resistance to medical management 80
rewards 87
in pot training 30
rhythmical activity 77
ricinoleic acid 66
running away 90
Ruysch, Fredick 3

sabotage 84, 87, 90
sacral plexus 6
saline cathartics 65
scapegoat 87
Schwann cell bundles 72
scoliosis 46
secondary constipation 42–3
secrecy 57
secret bucket 85
self esteem 89
low in neurogenic rectum 47
senna 62, 67–8
and anal pain 32
and spinal lesions 53
use, incidence 34
Senokot, see senna
sensation 12
and megarectum 37, 38
Avicenna's theory 65
rectal during anorectal manometry
77
sensory
innervation 9
receptors 9

separation from family 90
sex difference
with abdominal pain 41
with constipation 33
sexual abuse 91
Shakespeare 68
shame 83, 90
shaming 86
smooth muscle hypertrophy 41
Soavé 81
soiling 83
and abuse 91
and global developmental delay
44
and megarectum 39, 40
definition 1
incidence 33
survival packs 85
Soranus 2
spasticity 46
speech delay incidence 34
sphincterotomy 63, 81
for Hirschsprung's disease 23
for megarectum 39
sphincters
anal 6, 7
rectosigmoid 40
spina bifida 70
spina bifida occulta 70
spinal
dysraphism 70
lesions and neurogenic bowel 47–56
tumours 43
star chart 87
Starling's Law 38
Stevens–Johnson syndrome 66
stimulant laxatives 66–8
straining
and megarectum 40
and spinal lesions 51
stress 57, 88
stressors 84
stretch receptors 12
strictures, anorectal 19
structured approach 86
success rate, anal dilatation 80
suctional rectal biopsy 72
support
for child and family 85
to professionals 86
suppositories
inappropriate 13, 31
use, incidence 34